Improving Discipline-Based Undergraduate Medical Curriculum

Kadambari D • Kumar S
Zayapragassarazan Z • Parija SC

Improving Discipline-Based Undergraduate Medical Curriculum

An Evidence Informed Approach

Springer

Kadambari D
Department of Medical Education
Jawaharlal Institute of Postgraduate Medical Education and Research (JIPMER)
Puducherry
India

Kumar S
Department of Medical Education
Jawaharlal Institute of Postgraduate Medical Education and Research (JIPMER)
Puducherry
India

Zayapragassarazan Z
Department of Medical Education
Jawaharlal Institute of Postgraduate Medical Education and Research (JIPMER)
Puducherry
India

Parija SC
Former Director and Senior Professor of Microbiology
Jawaharlal Institute of Postgraduate Medical Education and Research (JIPMER)
Puducherry
India

ISBN 978-981-13-1309-7   ISBN 978-981-13-1310-3 (eBook)
https://doi.org/10.1007/978-981-13-1310-3

Library of Congress Control Number: 2018949154

This Springer imprint is published by the registered company Springer Nature Singapore Pte Ltd.
The registered company address is: 152 Beach Road, #21-01/04 Gateway East, Singapore 189721, Singapore

Preface

Discipline-based undergraduate curriculum is a widely used curriculum for undergraduate medical education across the world. However, there have been criticisms levelled against discipline-based approach and several of its deficiencies have been pointed out. One of the shortcomings cited is that the product of such a curriculum is insufficiently equipped to meet the challenges of current healthcare needs. One of the reasons may be that the teaching of basic sciences tends to go beyond what is needed by the undergraduate medical students for understanding and practicing primary health care. As a consequence, many strategies have been proposed. One of the strategies currently in vogue is the outcomes-based approach wherein the exit behaviours of a medical graduate are explicitly laid down and are used to guide the educational process. The shortcomings present in discipline-based undergraduate medical curriculum can be overcome by the strengths of these strategies. In this book we recommend improving discipline-based undergraduate medical curriculum with the help of a combination of several strategies including the adoption of outcomes-based approach and the use of evidence-informed implementable solutions. It is also recommended that support systems including educational leadership, curriculum committee, faculty development, student support, educational environment and programme evaluation should be given due emphasis for effective planning and implementation of changes in undergraduate medical curriculum.

The main reason for writing this book is to make available in one volume important strategies which can be used to improve discipline-based undergraduate medical curriculum. We have tried to present the message in an easy-to-understand way. We hope that faculty, administrators and policy makers will find the book useful. This can also be used as a resource for faculty development programmes.

We thank Springer Nature team for their support and guidance in the preparation of the manuscript and the book. We acknowledge the excellent artwork of Mr. Y. Kannan, Artist, JIPMER, for the preparation of cartoons. We also acknowledge the valuable assistance of Mr. D. Dhanasekarin, Data Entry Operator, JIPMER, in the typesetting and formatting of the manuscript.

PY, India — Kadambari D
PY, India — Kumar S
PY, India — Zayapragassarazan Z
PY, India — Parija SC

Contents

Part III Improving Discipline-based Undergraduate Medical Curriculum

About the Authors

Kadambari D works as a professor in the Department of Surgery at Jawaharlal Institute of Postgraduate Medical Education and Research (JIPMER), Puducherry, India. She also heads the Department of Medical Education at JIPMER. She completed the FAIMER-Keele Master of Health Professions Education (MHPE) and was awarded the MHPE.

She has participated and conducted on-site and off-site training programmes for teachers in the health profession including faculty, nurse educators and senior residents and the revised basic course workshops of the Medical Council of India (MCI) as Convener of the MCI Regional Centre for Faculty Development Programmes. She is currently the coordinator for curriculum reform of the MBBS course at JIPMER. She has also contributed to developing programmes of health education for the public on various aspects of health and disease and has taken part in conducting and organising health awareness camps particularly in the field of oncology. Her area of interest in surgery is breast surgery and particularly in oncoplastic breast surgery for breast cancer.

Kumar S presently works as technical consultant in the Department of Medical Education at Jawaharlal Institute of Postgraduate Medical Education and Research (JIPMER). Prior to this, Dr. Kumar has been head of the Department of Medical Education and Department of Urology, project officer and core group faculty member of National Teacher Training Centre (NTTC), JIPMER. He has organised, coordinated and functioned as a resource person in educational activities of the department including national courses on educational science for teachers of health professionals and integrated orientation programmes for interns and postgraduate students. Dr. Kumar has also been a resource person for on-site and off-site workshops on training of trainers, educational technology for residents, curriculum development, research methodology and biomedical research communication, Medical Council of India's basic course workshops in medical education technologies and one-day sensitization programmes on attitude and communication module.

Dr. Kumar has been the editor of the *Indian Journal of Urology*. Dr. Kumar has been the recipient of the WHO fellowship in the Institute of Urology, London, UK. Dr. Kumar has published several books, chapters and articles in medical education and in urology.

Zayapragassarazan Z presently works as additional professor in the Department of Medical Education at Jawaharlal Institute of Postgraduate Medical Education and Research (JIPMER), Puducherry, India. He was awarded Ph.D. in educational technology. He has published research and thematic articles in scientific and educational journals and contributed to books on education with reference to Indian context. He has presented papers in international and national conferences. He has introduced emerging areas of medical education such as active learning methods, e-learning, interactive teaching, teaching of attitude and communication skills through faculty development programmes organised in JIPMER. He currently serves as the co-convener of the MCI Regional Centre for Faculty Development Programmes. He is an advanced trauma life support (ATLS®) educator in India for ATLS® instructor course developed by the American College of Surgeons. He is a life member of several professional associations. He has served as resource person for University Grants Commission (UGC). Dr. Z. Zayapragassarazan was awarded the Broad Outlook Learner Teacher (BOLT) Award by Air India in 2006 and FAIMER fellowship in 2015. He is an approved research guide for PhD in Medical Education Technologies.

Parija SC is former Director and Senior Professor of Microbiology at Jawaharlal Institute of Postgraduate Medical Education and Research (JIPMER), Pondicherry, India, and has nearly three and half decades of teaching and research experience in medical microbiology. Prof. Parija is a Food and Agriculture Organization (FAO) expert and has been consulted to draft guidelines on food safety for parasites. He was on the board of MD examination at Colombo University, Sri Lanka; Sultan Qaboos University, Oman; and University of Malaya, Malaysia. He was conferred a D.Sc. for his contributions in the field of medical parasitology by Madras University. The author of ten books including the *Text Book of Medical Parasitology*, he has published more than 300 papers in both national and international journals of repute.

Prof. Parija has been honoured with more than 25 awards including the Medical Council of India's Dr. BC Roy National Award and the National Academy of Medical Sciences' Dr. PN Chuttani Oration Award. Prof. Parija founded the Indian Academy of Tropical Parasitology (IATP), the only professional organisation of medical parasitologists in India, and initiated the journal *Tropical Parasitology*.

Part I

An Appraisal of Discipline-Based Undergraduate Medical Curriculum

1 Appraising the Curriculum

Objectives

1. Define discipline-based undergraduate medical curriculum.
2. Describe the strengths of discipline-based undergraduate medical curriculum.
3. Discuss the limitations of discipline-based undergraduate medical curriculum.

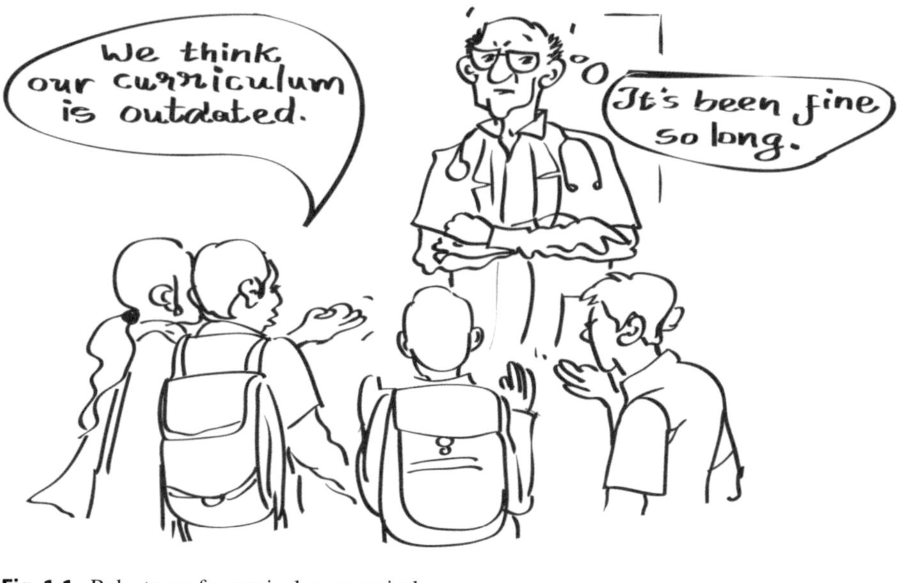

Fig. 1.1 Reluctance for curriculum appraisal

Kadambari D et al., *Improving Discipline-Based Undergraduate Medical Curriculum*, https://doi.org/10.1007/978-981-13-1310-3_1

1.1 Introduction

Discipline-based undergraduate medical curriculum is defined as a curriculum in which courses are identified by the names of disciplines such as anatomy, physiology, pathology, pharmacology, etc. in the first 2 years or in preclinical and paraclinical phases of the programme (Hecker and Violato 2008). In a typical discipline-based curriculum, curriculum is organized around disciplines, content is controlled by departments and teaching method is lecture (Papa and Harasym 1999). Discipline-based approach was introduced in North America in 1871 following similar practice in Germany and France (Papa and Harasym 1999). In the study of Hecker and Violato (2008), the use of discipline-based approach was reported by 65.5% medical schools of the United States in 1992 and by 40.5% medical schools in 1999. Discipline-based approach has remained the commonest in undergraduate medical education in India (Supe and Burdick 2006). In this chapter, the strengths and limitations of discipline-based undergraduate medical curriculum are described.

1.2 Strengths of Discipline-Based Undergraduate Medical Curriculum

Discipline-based undergraduate medical curriculum has the following strengths.

1.2.1 Existing Discipline-Based Departmental Organization

Discipline-based curriculum requires discipline-based organization. Discipline-based departmental organization already exists in medical schools. Thus existing discipline-based departmental organization can be used for delivering discipline-based undergraduate medical curriculum. This obviates any need for having another organizational and administrative setup (Reynolds III et al. 1995).

1.2.2 Teaching of Fundamentals of Disciplines

Fundamentals of disciplines involved in undergraduate medical education can be taught by subject experts. This teaching is aligned to the main purpose of the disciplines (Reynolds III et al. 1995). Teaching of fundamentals of these disciplines is required to enable students to pursue postgraduate programmes in any of the disciplines later.

1.3 Limitations of Discipline-Based Undergraduate Medical Curriculum

The limitations of discipline-based undergraduate medical curriculum are described under the following groups.

1.3.1 Factual Information Overload

Learning can either be with understanding or without understanding by rote. Learning with understanding is always preferable to learning by rote. According to the view of constructivism (Kaufman 2003) learning with understanding requires engagement of learners for reflecting on information to be learnt and relating this information to their existing knowledge. The cognitive activities of reflecting and relating require sufficient time. If there is too much information to learn and sufficient time is not available, students abandon constructivist approach and resort to learning by rote (Harden and Davis 1995). This state in which the amount of information exceeds the cognitive capacity for processing it for understanding can be called information overload (Kumar and Maskara 2015). As most of information overload in undergraduate discipline-based curriculum occurs due to factual information, it is also called factual overload (Harden and Davis 1995). Memorized information is forgotten unless it is regularly used (Harden et al. 1984). Factual overload is caused by the primacy given to covering the course in various disciplines and not to achieving the goals of MBBS programme. Factual information overload (Harden et al. 1984; Reynolds III et al. 1995; Papa and Harasym 1999) has been a long-standing problem in undergraduate medical curriculum as evidenced by the following quotations.

> As far back as 1863 a tendency to an overloading of the curriculum of education … followed by results injurious to the student was noted with concern ….
>
> General Medical Council (1993)

> Notwithstanding these repeated exhortations, there remains gross overcrowding of most undergraduate curricula, acknowledged by teachers and deplored by students.
>
> General Medical Council (1993)

> It is a common perception that the syllabus is excessively theoretical, making it difficult for the fresh graduate to effectively meet even the primary health care needs of the population.
>
> Govt. of India, National Health Policy (2002)

With continuing information explosion in all disciplines of medical science and with continuing improvement of information and communication technology, more information is likely to be more available in the future. With increasing information, the problem of factual information overload in discipline-based undergraduate medical curriculum/programme is likely to increase unless some measure is taken to define information needs.

1.3.2 Isolated Learning and Assessment

In discipline-based undergraduate medical curriculum, disciplines are taught in isolation independent of other disciplines (Harden et al. 1984; Reynolds III et al. 1995; Papa and Harasym 1999). Isolated teaching of disciplines without interrelating ideas with those of other disciplines may promote rote learning. Memorized information without regular use may be forgotten (Harden et al. 1984). Isolated teaching of disciplines can also lead to unnecessary repetitions, inclusion of irrelevant areas and contradictions of concepts. Due to fragmented disciplinary teaching, students have to integrate most of the learning on their own (Papa and Harasym 1999). Isolated assessment of students in various disciplines may also promote fragmented learning.

1.3.3 Teacher-Centred Approach

In teacher-centred approach, the focus is on teachers and their teaching in contrast to student-centred approach in which the focus is on students and their learning (Harden et al. 1984). In teacher-centred approach, teachers decide everything about the curriculum with little or no participation of students. In discipline-based undergraduate medical curriculum, teacher-centred approach is used. Teacher-controlled teaching-learning methods (Indira Gandhi National Open University 1991) are also associated with discipline-based undergraduate curriculum. Teacher-controlled methods include lecture, tutorial, team teaching, practical demonstration and bedside clinic which usually have low or medium student engagement. Student-/learner-controlled teaching-learning methods (Indira Gandhi National Open University 1991) include a small group discussion and individual learning methods (assignment, project, oral presentation, e-learning, skills lab learning, portfolio, OSCE/OSPE). Student-controlled methods, which usually have high student engagement and use constructivist approach to learning, are seldom used in discipline-based undergraduate curriculum.

As lecture is the most efficient teacher-controlled method for transmission of information, it is commonly a preferred method. Student-controlled methods listed above can also be used for assessment. Teacher-centred approach also has the limitation of having rigid timetables and lacking academic flexibility. Students also do not have any choice of learning things of their interest as there are no electives.

1.3.4 Opportunistic Clinical Teaching-Learning

In traditional discipline-based undergraduate medical curriculum, students are posted in departments by rotation. Students study cases which are selected from cases available at that time in wards or outpatient department. Thus, teaching-learning is mostly opportunistic (Harden et al. 1984). It is possible that by chance all students in various batches may not be able to study educationally required numbers of cases of educationally required clinical presentations and diseases. All students may not be able to achieve all necessary outcomes/competencies which is educationally not acceptable.

1.3.5 Neglect of MBBS Programme Goals

MBBS programme has its goals expressed in outcome frameworks such as the roles of an Indian Medical Graduate including clinician, leader and member of the health-care team and system, communicator, lifelong learner and professional (Medical Council of India's Regulations on Graduate Medical Education-Proposed 2012) and CanMEDS Physician Competency Framework (Canada) including medical expert, communicator, collaborator, leader, health advocate, scholar and professional (Frank et al. 2015). These roles, competencies and other important areas such as behavioural sciences, evidence-informed medicine and patient safety are neglected in discipline-based undergraduate medical curriculum/programme because responsibility and accountability for education in these areas, roles and competencies are not assigned explicitly. Thus in discipline-based undergraduate curriculum, the purpose of MBBS programme is not emphasized (Reynolds III et al. 1995).

1.3.6 Resistance to Change

In discipline-based undergraduate medical curriculum/programme, the departments of disciplines and their teachers control the content and teaching-learning programme (Papa and Harasym 1999). There is resistance to change for improving undergraduate curriculum/programme (Reynolds III et al. 1995) because the affinity for disciplines is usually more than that for MBBS programme.

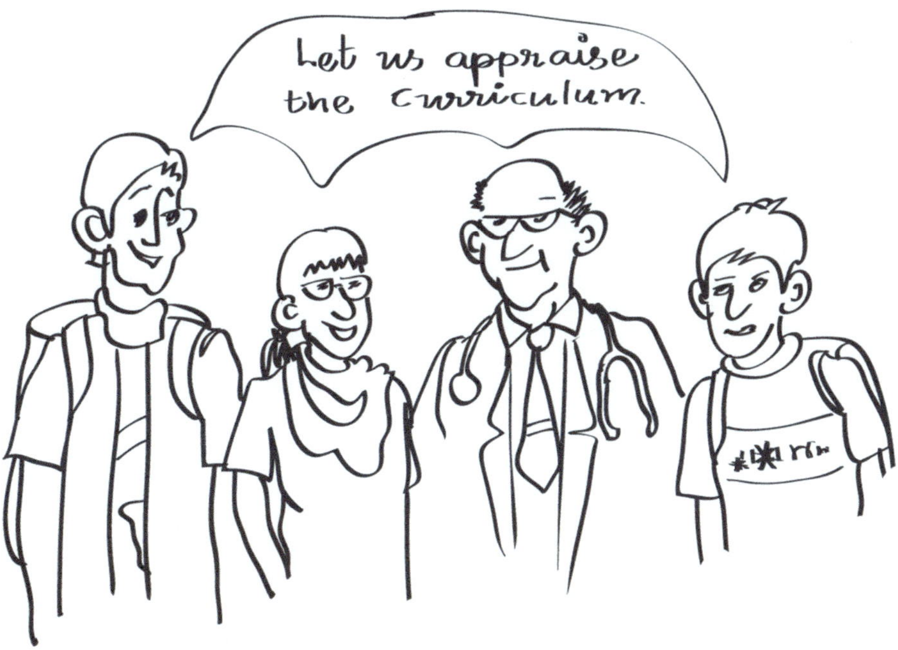

Fig. 1.2 Acceptance of curriculum appraisal

Conclusions

The strengths of discipline-based undergraduate medical curriculum include existing discipline-based departmental organization and teaching of fundamentals of disciplines by subject experts. The limitations of discipline-based undergraduate medical curriculum include factual information overload, isolated learning and assessment, teacher-centred approach, opportunistic clinical teaching-learning, neglect of MBBS programme goals and resistance to change. Regular updating of discipline-based undergraduate medical curriculum should address these limitations.

References

Frank JR, Snell L, Sherbino J (eds) (2015) CanMEDS 2015 physician competency framework. Royal College of Physicians and Surgeons of Canada, Ottawa Available from www.royalcollege.ca/rcsite/documents/canmeds/canmeds-full-framework-e.pdf. Accessed 8 Jan 2018

General Medical Council (1993) Tomorrow's Doctors. Recommendations on Undergraduate Medical Education.

Government of India. National Health Policy (2002) Ministry of Health and Family Welfare, Government of India; 2002. Available from https://childlineindia.org.in/CP-CR-Downloads/National_Health_policy_2002.pdf. Accessed 13 Jan 2018

Harden RM, Davis MH (1995) AMEE Medical Education Guide No 5. The core curriculum with options or special study modules. Med Teach 17(2):125–148 Available from https://amee.org/getattachment/AMEE-Initiatives/ESME-Courses/AMEE-ESME-Face-to-Face-Courses/ESME/ESME-Online-Resources-China-Dec-2015/AMEE-Guide-No-5.PDF. Accessed 13 Jan 2018

Harden RM, Sowden S, Dunn WR (1984) Educational strategies in curriculum development: the SPICES model. Med Educ 18:284–297 Available from https://amee.org/getattachment/AMEE-Initiatives/ESME-Courses/AMEE-ESME-Face-to-Face-Courses/ESME/ESME-Online-Resources-China-Dec-2015/The-SPICES-Model.pdf. Accessed 13 Jan 2018

Hecker K, Violato C (2008) How much do differences in medical schools influence student performance? A longitudinal study employing hierarchical linear modeling. Teach Learn Med 20(2):104–113. https://doi.org/10.1080/10401330801991915

Indira Gandhi National Open University (1991) Instruction in a systemic perspective. In: ES-302 instruction in higher education. PGDHE course material. Indira Gandhi National Open University, New Delhi, pp 27–60

Kaufman DM (2003) Applying educational theory in practice. In: Cantillon P, Hutchinson L, Wood D (eds) ABC of learning and teaching in medicine. BMJ Publishing Group, London, pp 1–4

Kumar A, Maskara S (2015) Coping up with the information overload in the medical profession. J Biosc Med 3:124–127. https://doi.org/10.4236/jbm.2015.311016

Medical Council of India. Regulations on Graduate Medical Education-Proposed (2012) Available from http://iafmonline.in/data/circular-notifications/Revised-GME-2012.pdf. Accessed 8 Jan 2018

Papa FJ, Harasym PH (1999) Medical curriculum reform in North America, 1765 to the present: a cognitive science perspective. Acad Med 74(2):154–164 PMID: 10065057.Available from https://www.ncbi.nlm.nih.gov/pubmed/10065057. Accessed 13 Jan 2018

Reynolds CF III, Adler S, Kanter SL, Horn JP, Harvey J, Bernier GM Jr (1995) The undergraduate medical curriculum: centralized versus departmentalized. Acad Med 70(8):671–675 Available from http://journals.lww.com/academicmedicine/abstract/1995/08000/the_undergraduate_medical_curriculum__centralized.7.aspx. Accessed 13 Jan 2018

Supe A, Burdick WP (2006) Challenges and issues in medical education in India. Acad Med 81(12):1076–1080. https://doi.org/10.1097/01.ACM.0000246699.94234.ab PMID: 17122473.

Part II

Research and Evidence in Education for Improving Discipline-based Undergraduate Medical Curriculum

2 Using Research and Evidence

Objectives
After reading this chapter, the reader would be able to:

1. Understand the role of research in curriculum improvement.
2. Appreciate the differences between educational and biomedical research.
3. Become familiar with the paradigms and approaches to research in education.
4. Appraise and use findings from quantitative and qualitative research studies in education.

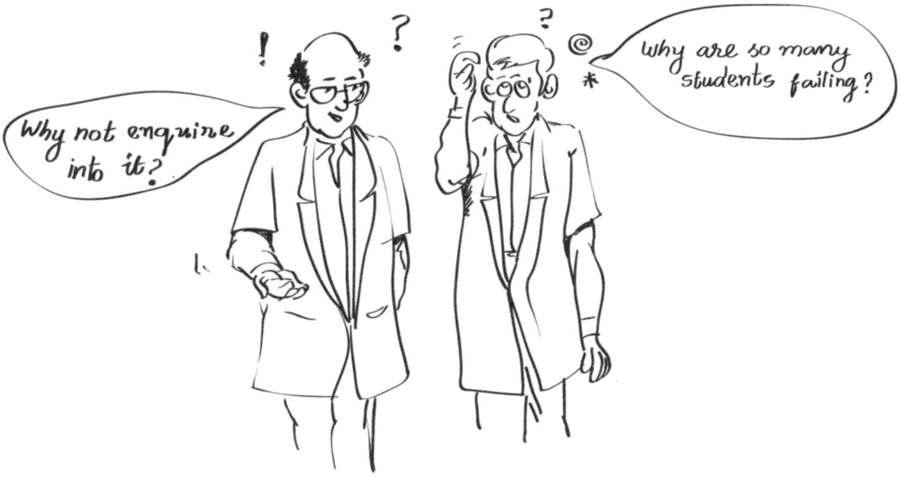

Fig. 2.1 The need for research in education

Kadambari D et al., *Improving Discipline-Based Undergraduate Medical Curriculum*, https://doi.org/10.1007/978-981-13-1310-3_2

Curriculum improvement is a continuous process involving a regular, timely appraisal of existing practice and implementing changes that have a rational basis. Continuous evaluation provides the data regarding the performance of the curriculum and highlights areas that need improvement. For changes to have a rational basis, they should be supported by sufficient evidence. This chapter provides the reader with a broad understanding of the various research methods in education and ways of using the findings of such research to improve the curriculum.

2.1 What Is Evidence in Education?

Evidence may be defined as 'the available body of facts or information indicating whether a belief or proposition is true or valid' (Oxford Dictionary).

Evidence may be gathered from facts that are available (logical evidence), from research (empirical evidence) or from individual experience (anecdotal evidence). Different types of evidence serve different purposes (Thistlethwaite et al. 2012).

Research evidence obtained by analysis of a mass of data and observations already made could result in the development of a theory. With the help of research, one can 'obtain evidence to support or refute proposed facts or principles' (Fraenkel et al. 2011). Alternately, a hypothesis may be framed on the basis of existing data and an experiment conducted to test the facts. This provides a means of gathering empirical evidence from research.

In medical practice the move towards evidence-based practice/evidence-based medicine (EBM) began in the 1990s. Evidence-based medicine has been defined as 'the conscientious, explicit, and judicious use of current best evidence in making decisions about the care of individual patients' with the implicit assertion that data are superior to authority and tradition (Sackett et al. 1996). It is recognized, however, that the proficiency and judgement of the clinician obtained from experience and practice are important in assessing the applicability of evidence to her practice.

Extrapolating this principle to education, there has been a consistent call to improve educational policy and practice on the basis of sound evidence from scientific research (Tranfield et al. 2003; Lemons et al. 2014). When designing instruction, taking into consideration the 'science of learning' (Mayer 2010) provides a sound basis for choice of the instructional method, for example, on how to use a judicious mix of verbal and visual learning resources. At a macrolevel (Levinson 2010), as in curriculum development, large amounts of time and effort and resources are invested in making policy changes. Also, as educators of future health professionals, we are accountable to the healthcare system and to society at large. Our decisions, therefore, must be backed by sound principles and the best available evidence obtained from well-conducted systematic research rather than on opinion.

In our day-to-day practice as teachers of health professionals, we encounter challenges including holding students' attention in a lecture, guiding them when performing tricky practical procedures and measuring the level of their learning. We may turn to our prior experience for a solution or discuss our problems with more experienced peers, either of which strategies may give us a solution, but we don't often look to research evidence for the answer.

Davies (1999) describes the role of educationalists in the practice of evidence-informed education as twofold. The first role is in *using* the evidence, whereby an educationalist poses questions about education, systematically looks for and finds the evidence, weighs it and decides on its relevance; the other role is to *establish* the evidence, whereby the educationalist plans and carries out studies of high scientific rigour in order to establish sound evidence where such is lacking. In education, too, as in clinical medicine, the professional judgement of the individual teacher is needed to determine the applicability of the evidence to her context.

However, evidence in education is not easily defined or obtained. Education is a social science, and research in the social sciences are value driven and look for meanings of phenomena in contrast to research in the natural sciences which are focused on establishing causality, viewing the world as external and science as value-free. Educational experiments deal with humans who show a highly individualized response to interventions. This compounded by the large number of variables that are peculiar to the context of the experiment makes the results poorly generalizable. For example, an experiment that tests whether intervention A resulted in better conceptual understanding among learners (as determined by performance on standardized tests) than what is being done at present will encounter the confounders brought in by the variable level of prior knowledge among the students, the level of motivation among the learners, the acceptability of the new intervention, teacher factors such as level of experience, familiarity with the intervention and so on. And if we do adjust for these confounding factors by choosing a highly selective group of learners and teachers, the results would be less generalizable. Biomedical research experiments adjust for variability by selecting random and large samples and using mathematical measures to establish cause and effect. Such research attempts to answer the question 'Does it work?' with the primary purpose of generalizing the results to other contexts and populations. Would this mean that randomization and using large samples provide generalizable results in educational research? Not really. Randomization is applicable in very few situations in educational research. For example, curriculum studies cannot be randomized. 'Blinding' which is very often employed in biomedical experiments is virtually impossible in education.

How then do we adopt findings from research done in other contexts and situations into our practice? The answer is 'We probably shouldn't!' at least not without testing it in our local situation with its contextual (social, economic, political) factors and with our learners who have unique attributes. What we can do in educational research is look for explanations and meanings to generate theory and conduct experiments in different contexts that would support or challenge the theory.

Thistlethwaite et al. (2012) argue that there is no one 'metadefinition' of evidence in medical education. Instead they espouse a more pluralistic approach to defining evidence with consideration of its purpose, the source, the stakeholders and its relationship to theory. Thus evidence derived using statistical calculations from experimental studies is *probably* true and may be generalizable to other settings, while with narrative reasoning, evidence that is *plausibly* true for an individual case can be obtained. A *realist* perspective blends the two viewpoints to produce 'evidence on what generally works for whom, most of the time and given certain contextual preconditions' (Thistlethwaite et al. 2012). One must also remember that research produces inanimate data, which must be set in context and interpreted by a human mind taking other knowledge and data into consideration in order to be used as evidence that is meaningful enough for taking action. Therefore, production of knowledge from research is a 'deeply social and contextual process'.

Harden et al. (1999) emphasizes the importance of having evidence before introducing a new practice in education—evidence that 'confirms the value of the intervention'. Relevant evidence may come from research and from professional experience of teachers and could also be based on theory or educational principles.

Research can inform practice in one of two ways. It can be the source of instrumental knowledge (technical role) that provides information on what one should do in order to achieve an outcome. Thus research provides practitioners with knowledge about 'what works', for example, effective strategies for teaching, assessment or for supporting learning. Research also has a cultural role, that is, it provides different interpretations and understanding of educational practice (Biesta 2007).

Much has been done in the field of education since Plato and Aristotle. There are learning theories from the field of education psychology that attempt to explain how learning occurs, help teachers solve educational problems, improve their teaching strategies or understand what goes on in the minds of learners. Although mostly from general and school education, much of it is applicable in medical education. Equipping medical teachers with the principles of educational psychology will certainly help them to practice their skills in a better, more informed way. There are also publications of educational experiments conducted in different settings that provide some information on whether or not a particular educational intervention worked in a particular setting. There are also publications of research that have attempted to explain phenomena or describe contextual experiences.

However, one must not expect research findings to provide instant solutions to problems in the field. The findings must be contextualized, judged whether useful and then tried, tested and adopted in a suitably adapted form. Professional knowledge and experience have significant influence on how research findings are interpreted. One must also take care to remember that 'evidence is what the powerful say it is' (Thistlethwaite et al. 2012). As educators in our own right, we must be able to critically appraise research and avoid blindly adopting practices that have been espoused by 'big names' in the field.

Davies (1999) stresses the importance of the need to integrate the individual teacher's expertise with best available external evidence from research and defines evidence-based education as:

> ...a set of principles and practices which can alter the way people can think about education, the way they go about educational policy and the basis on which they make their professional judgement and deploy their expertise.

Harden et al. (1999) describe a continuum of practice with 100% opinion-based teaching at the left end and 100% evidence-based teaching at the right end. The teacher would find herself closer to either end depending on whether or not a significant body of evidence is available for decision-making.

2.2 Educational Research

2.2.1 Paradigms and Approaches

Taylor and Medina (2013) define a paradigm (from Greek 'para' = beside and 'deigma' = example) as a 'comprehensive belief system, a worldview or a framework that guides research and practice in a field'. Paradigms are 'theoretical frameworks' adopted as a world view. A research paradigm comprises a view of reality (ontology), a view of the knowledge generated (epistemology) and the approach to generating that knowledge (methodology). Paradigms 'act as lenses through which scientists or researchers are able to perceive and understand the problems in their field and the scientific answers to their problems' (Hathaway 1995).

Lukenchuk and Kolich (2013) identify six paradigms in educational research for the twenty-first century, namely, empirical-analytical, pragmatic, interpretive, critical, post-structuralist and transcendental. They emphasize that choosing the appropriate paradigm(s) for a research project is the key to its successful planning, including the selection of appropriate methodologies and the project's subsequent implementation.

Shifts in paradigms accompanied changing ideas about knowledge, moving away from a positivist stance with its stress on verifiability to pragmatism and interpretivism and a critical approach to the idea of knowledge. Today, research can be described as being multiparadigmatic (Hammersley 2012).

The approaches to generation of new knowledge by research include quantitative, qualitative and mixed methods (Anshu and Grant 2014).

The *quantitative approach* consists of studies that draw conclusions with statistical reasoning. The aim of quantitative research is to look at 'cause-effect' relationships and to answer the question 'Does this (intervention) work?' It aims at the replicability and generalizability of the results obtained from a study conducted on a random sample of the population under investigation. Study designs commonly included under this approach include surveys, assessments, experimental and quasi-experimental studies, correlational studies and so on (Cleland and Jamieson 2014). Although it can be argued that true generalizability is questionable as the results are derived from only a sample of a large population of interest, the errors due to sampling are minimized by random selection, using large samples and with the use of statistical calculations. Study methods used in quantitative research include questionnaires, rating scales, psychometric tests and psychological tests. A main characteristic of quantitative studies is their 'objectivity' with the researcher staying 'outside' the study setting.

The quantitative approach does not explain *why* something occurs. Explanations of phenomena and the effects of human behaviour and interactions are not addressed by quantitative studies. With the *qualitative approach*, 'the researcher tries to make sense of how others see the world' (Stewart and Filice de Barros 2014). In contrast to quantitative research which deals with numbers, qualitative approaches use words as sources of data. The researcher aims to view the issue under research from the participant's eyes and is herself an 'insider' to the research process, with her own thoughts, ideas and feelings influencing the interpretation of the data. Sampling is usually purposive, and sample sizes are usually smaller than in quantitative studies. The type of sampling used in qualitative research varies with the purpose of the study. The research could include only the most usual cases of the phenomenon under study (typical case sampling) or only the extreme cases of the phenomenon (deviant case sampling) or include only cases that are particularly information rich (critical case sampling) or a wide range of cases to include typical, critical and deviant cases to capture the broadest set of information and experiences (maximum variation sampling). The sample may consist of individuals whose perspectives are likely to confirm (confirming sampling) or challenge (disconfirming sampling) the researcher's developing understanding of the phenomenon (Kuper et al. 2008). The results of qualitative studies, therefore, are locally relevant to the particular sample of participants and are not usually generalizable to other situations. Qualitative studies can be seen as hypothesis-generating rather than hypothesis-testing.

Research designs used in qualitative research projects include:

1. Phenomenology—this refers to the study of phenomena and focuses on the subjective experience of the individual; phenomenological studies do not necessarily provide explanations but raise awareness and increase insight, focusing on the meaning human beings make of their experience (van der Mescht 2004). For example, how do clinician faculty describe their experience with teaching during bedside clinics?
2. Grounded theory—grounded theory focuses on theory generation about phenomena. The purpose of grounded theory research is to build a theoretical model of how a process or action works (Chen and Teherani 2016). Data collection and analysis proceed simultaneously each informing the other (Watling and Lingard 2012). For example, how do students learn during bedside teaching sessions? How does role modelling impact their learning?
3. Ethnography—this has a background in anthropology and means 'portrait of a people'. It is used to conduct descriptive studies of cultures and people. Ethnographic research is time-consuming as it goes beyond simply describing details of a particular event (MacLeod 2016) and seeks to explain them from a cultural perspective, that is, an insider's view. The characteristic of ethnography is the presentation of study findings as what are termed 'thick descriptions', that is, the description of behaviours of people and places being studied is made more meaningful to the reader of the research by the inclusion of explanations of the settings/context where the study has taken place (Reeves et al. 2013). For exam-

ple, what is the experience of first year undergraduate learners in the first 2 months of medical school?

4. Case study—this design is used to describe, in depth, a single unit such as a person, an organization or an institution. Some studies describe a series of cases. Studies range in complexity from illustrative descriptions of single events to extended studies that trace events involving the same participants over a period of time. Case studies are aimed to provide in-depth detailed description of one particular case; hence, it is left to the reader of the research findings to judge its representativeness to their own local situation. For example, what factors influence curriculum change from a traditional discipline-based approach to an integrated one at X medical school?
5. Critical theory—the goal of critical theory is emancipation of the oppressed. Its purpose is to critique and challenge with the intention of introducing social change (Stewart and Filice de Barros 2014).

Data collection methods in qualitative research include interviews, focus group discussions, observations and textual analysis. Interviews may be structured, that is, the questions are predetermined and are uniformly asked of all participants. Alternatively, they may be semi-structured or unstructured where a few or all questions, respectively, allow for participants' responses to steer the interview in a direction that is not predetermined. Unstructured interviews are also termed in-depth interviews.

Focus group discussions are appropriate when group interactions are needed to obtain deeper insights or when resources are insufficient for interviewing individual participants (for more information on conducting focus group discussions, see Stalmeijer et al. 2014).

Observations are used when it is not necessary to interact with people. The observed entity may be people, the environment they are in, as in an ethnographic study of certain ethnic groups. Data are in the form of written observations, video recordings or photographs or other artefacts and documentation such as policy documents, annual reports, minutes of meetings and so on.

Mixed method research refers to the adoption of a research strategy employing more than one type of research method (Brannen 2005). These could be combinations of quantitative and qualitative methods or the use of more than one quantitative method or more than one qualitative method. It could also refer to the use of different types of data or that there are several research teams working in different research paradigms.

There have been heated debates among education researchers over the degree to which quantitative and qualitative methods can be combined. There are three perspectives which researchers may fall into—*purists*, who assert the incommensurability of the two approaches; *situationalists*, who choose the most appropriate methods for specific situations alternating between quantitative and qualitative methodologies; and the *pragmatist* to whom the two approaches can be used together throughout the research, combining the strengths of both approaches (Hathaway 1995).

The purpose of combining the results from different data analysis includes:

1. Corroboration/triangulation—different methods check or validate one another.
2. Elaboration—one type of data adds to the understanding being gained by another.
3. Initiation—one method raises hypotheses or research questions to be pursued by another method.
4. Complementarity—each type of data analysis enhances the other.
5. Contradiction—when findings are in conflict and may lead to discounting one method in favour of the other following assessments of validity and reliability.

The first step in deciding on the research strategy is to determine the logic of inquiry—whether inductive or deductive. Many projects involve both, for example, a survey. If a mixed method approach is the logic, the ordering of methods must be determined, whether sequential or simultaneous. The next step is to determine which one would be the dominant form, in terms of resource allocation. The commonest combination is when a qualitative pilot work is precedent to a large survey (larger resource allocation). Mixed method research also incorporates the flexibility to alter the methods during the study.

2.2.2 Syntheses of Educational Research

Patrício and vaz Carneiro (2012) define evidence-based education as 'the methodology by which educationalists and other teaching professionals including policy makers, managers, students etc., base their decisions to support medical education interventions'. Educational research asks complex questions that attempt to find answers to a multitude of issues, including policy and practice problems, causal pathways, interventions and their consequences, experiences of those exposed to the interventions and the complex processes of implementation and delivery (Dixon-Woods et al. 2005). These questions require complex forms of evidence. *Syntheses of research evidence* provide a means of putting together evidence obtained from several primary studies that all address a common research question. Systematic review is a type of research synthesis designed to support evidence-informed practice. Systematic reviews are a form of secondary research which originated in the social sciences spreading to medicine and now to medical education.

The argument in medicine is that as clinicians cannot keep pace with the changes occurring in their science, systematic reviews that summarize best practice are necessary to inform clinical decision-making (Clegg 2005). Typified by the Cochrane Reviews in clinical medicine, systematic reviews are described as syntheses of multiple primary investigations employing strategies to limit random error and bias. Thus systematic reviews in clinical medicine require the employment of rigorous and standardized procedures. Patrício and vaz Carneiro (2012) lists the following basic steps of a systematic review:

1. Formulating a clinically relevant question.
2. Explicit selection of studies to be included in the review.

3. Critical appraisal of the evidence.
4. Synthesis of the evidence.
5. Statistical analysis of the results.

Emphasizing the need for a sound evidence base for teaching, Harden et al. (1999) established the Best Evidence Medical Education (BEME) initiative on the principle 'In BEME the culture or ethos is such that teachers are encouraged to question their practice, to look for the best evidence available, to relate the evidence to their own situation and to apply their professional judgements'. The aim of BEME was to assist teachers to evaluate the evidence for relevance to their own practice. The BEME has now evolved into an international Best Evidence Medical and Health Professional Education collaboration between groups of health professional educators, universities and professional organizations, whose work has been described as 'an effort to move from the use of anecdotal information in medical education to the use of evidence synthesis through systematic review, mirroring the revolution seen in healthcare' (Gordon and Patricio 2016). The BEME collaboration provides organizational, scholarly and publication support to interested groups of reviewers including training opportunities in the form of seminars (Thistlethwaite and Hammick 2010).

One of the main purposes of a systematic review is to provide an unbiased recommendation for or against a particular intervention. This would require primary studies to be those conducted with sufficient rigour.

Often, the reviewers may inadvertently introduce bias in the selection of review criteria, the data abstraction process and the presentation of results. There may also be inherent biases in the studies being reviewed, which, if not taken into account, could result in a skewed statistical result (Cook 2008). Also, given the complex nature of educational research, there may be very few studies that would fulfil the rigorous inclusion and exclusion criteria listed for a systematic review, so that recommendations are often based on analysis of a handful of studies identified from among several thousand obtained from the initial 'scoping search'.

The place of systematic reviews in education has been a matter of much debate. In a critique of the practice of systematic reviews in education, MacLure (2005) argues that, in trying to provide statistically backed recommendations for or against an intervention, the richness of the data, that is, the value of the findings from the primary research, is undermined and describes this as 'a threat to quality and critique in scholarship and research'.

Eva (2008) highlights the difficulty of systematic reviews in education and instead recommends a critical narrative review of educational research which consists of 'a critical synthesis of a variety of literatures (and) identifies knowledge that is well established, highlights gaps in understanding, and provides some guidance regarding what remains to be understood'.

Rigour in educational research does not mean experimentation in tightly controlled conditions. Qualitative research also demands rigour in the methodology in order to provide answers and explanations. Systematic reviews often omit qualitative research evidence. This can have important consequences as some questions require a range of data sources to be examined.

Barnett-Page and Thomas (2009) describe several techniques for the synthesis of qualitative research studies.

1. Metaethnography—metaethnography aims at building understanding rather than merely aggregating data. The synthesis could comprise of developing overarching concepts by a process of reciprocal translational analysis, whereby similar concepts from individual studies are considered in the synthesis. Or it may involve the exploration and explanation of contradictions between individual studies (refutational synthesis). With a 'line of argument synthesis' approach, a picture of the whole (e.g. an organization) is created from studying its parts.
2. Grounded theory—this method synthesizes studies using the approach and principles of grounded theory research.
3. Thematic synthesis—combining the two approaches mentioned above, thematic synthesis consists of organizing the data into themes by identifying the commonality among studies. Hypothesis generation can result from this approach (Thomas and Harden 2008).
4. Textual narrative synthesis—this is used to synthesize studies of different types, e.g. qualitative and quantitative (Lucas et al. 2007). A standard format is followed for reporting on the study characteristics, context, findings and quality. The extracted data is then put into context with the help of structured summaries.
5. Meta-study—this is a multi-faceted approach comprising of analysis of findings (meta-data-analysis), analysis of methods (meta-methods) and analysis of theory (meta-theory) all of which may be conducted concurrently.
6. Meta-narrative—described by Greenhalgh et al. (2005), this approach is based on the principle that, across different paradigms, there are multiple ways of understanding the concept at the heart of a review. Studies from different research traditions are selected and their key features mapped.
7. Critical interpretive synthesis—Dixon-Woods et al. (2006) described this approach to the synthesis of multidisciplinary and multi-method studies. Adapting metaethnography, this method is also influenced by grounded theory in its inductive approach to the research question and the development of concepts and categories. The method has an 'explicit orientation towards theory generation'.
8. Ecological triangulation—this technique of research synthesis employs the principle of triangulation by which phenomena are studied from a variety of vantage points, with the resultant synthesis of cumulative multi-faceted evidence in order to find out 'what interventions work for what kind of outcomes for what kinds of persons under what kind of conditions' (Barnett-Page and Thomas 2009).
9. Framework synthesis—this is a method using a highly structured approach (e.g. with the use of numerical codes for indexing or using charts to depict data) that is used to analyse the large amounts of textual data that are obtained from qualitative studies.

Syntheses of qualitative evidence may not always be feasible and acceptable, especially with qualitative studies derived from different traditions and even when similar themes can be identified across all studies; the mixing of methods could lead to difficulties in developing theory.

Even more controversial is the attempt to synthesize qualitative with quantitative research and usually consists of converting all data into either quantitative or qualitative form for analysis. Techniques for these are, however, not very well described and rarely reported.

The nature of the research synthesis is ultimately decided by the question being asked. Dixon-Woods et al. (2005) categorize research synthesis into two overlapping methodologies, *integrative* and *interpretive.* Integrative synthesis focuses primarily on summarizing data that are generally well specified and seeks to establish causality and generalization rather than develop concepts. In contrast, interpretive synthesis, which is conceptual in its process and output, focuses on building theory while being grounded in the empirical data obtained from the studies.

It must be noted that, important as methodology and approach are, the epistemological (nature of knowledge) and ontological (understanding and perception of reality) orientations of the research are essential to determine the nature of the inquiry (Bunniss and Kelly 2010; Hathaway 1995). The appropriateness of the paradigm selected is far more critical to the quality of a research than the correctness of methods used.

The quantitative approach is orientated to the empirical-analytical paradigm with its positivistic leanings defining knowledge as objective, and the researcher remains 'detached' from the research setting.

In contrast, in the interpretive paradigm (qualitative approach), the experience of the human participant is central to the construction of reality and creation of knowledge. Interpretivism assumes that a study can never be bias-free (Bunniss and Kelly 2010) and the researcher's thoughts and feelings can influence her observations.

Thus in empirical-analytical research, generalizability seeks to develop universal knowledge, while, in the interpretive paradigm, the social context in which knowledge is gathered is the primary influence on its understanding.

The pragmatic paradigm is a problem-centred and action-oriented one, where truth is defined as the effectiveness of knowledge demonstrated by the effectiveness of action (Lukenchuk and Kolich 2013). Conceptually it has a strong link to the empirical-analytical paradigm and may be seen as an overarching paradigm that incorporates a variety of quantitative, qualitative and mixed method research projects.

2.2.3 Teacher as Researcher and the Place of Action Research

The central role of the teacher in educational research was emphasized by Stenhouse (1979) with his recommendation to use the classroom as a laboratory and 'in the command of the teachers, not researchers'. He defined research as a 'thoughtful study of problems' and promoted teacher-led inquiry based on *curiosity.* He challenged the concept of the teacher as authority and believed that teachers 'must be educated to develop their art, not master it, for the claim to mastery merely signals the abandoning of aspiration'. He reiterated the uncertainty of knowledge and the role of research in accumulating knowledge through the 'patient definition of error' and in strengthening the professional judgement of the teacher.

Action research has its origins in sociological studies in industrial settings (Adelman 1993).

McTaggart (1994) defines action research as:

> a form of collective, self-reflective enquiry undertaken by participants in social situations in order to improve the rationality and justice of their own social or educational practices, as well as their understanding of these practices and the situations in which these practices are carried out

Kurt Lewin is given the credit for being a major force behind action research. After World War II, he worked with the Commission on Community Interrelations in New York and worked on addressing prejudice and intergroup conflict. The commission's maxim was 'no research without action and no action without research'.

For Lewin, central to action research is the discussion of problems and group decisions on how to proceed. Thus, action research can be seen as a form of inquiry through which members of social groups (for instance, a group of teachers) 'interact with one another, engage in an open dialogue about their intergroup relationships and collectively participate in a learning process to create social change in their communities' (Glassman et al. 2013). Typically action research requires collaboration among all those who have a stake in the problem under investigation. This 'working together' by a community for the development of a social- or education-based intervention for a difficult problem is the core underpinning principle of action research.

There are four basic steps in action research (Fraenkal et al. 2011). It begins with framing the research question, gathering the required information, analysing it and devising a plan of action. The 'action' in action research begins with the collective challenging of rules and habits by the members of a community. The research question may be framed as 'What is the better way to teach cardiac physiology?' rather than as 'Is inquiry-based learning superior to traditional teaching for learning cardiac physiology?' The scope of action research, being practitioner initiated, is usually kept narrow, more complex research being left to researchers. Data gathered in action research may be any of the types collected in other forms of research and includes methodologies such as surveys, interviews, documentary analysis and ethnographies. The teacher herself may be an 'insider' or 'outsider' to the research. Analysis focuses on answering the 'why', 'what', 'who', 'how', 'when' and 'where' questions, the purpose of the analysis being to assess and make sense of the information gathered. The 'research' aspect of action research rests on open non-hierarchical dialogue between members all equally engaged in the process of change. It is important in action research therefore that all stakeholders (participants) be informed about the data and their inputs taken at the analysis stage rather than merely being informed about the results of the study. The final step is to create a plan of action to solve the problem identified, based on the findings. A formal report may or may not be prepared. What is essential is to have a clear direction of the next steps for implementing action.

The basic principle of action research is the active participation by the group in exploring the problems identified followed by decision-making, monitoring and noting the consequences with regular progress review. This constitutes the identify-plan-implement-evaluate cycle of action research. New problems identified during this process would again be brought in for discussion and action cycles—the 'action spiral'. This form of action inquiry describes any process that one follows in which action and inquiry into it lead to improvement of practice (Tripp 2005).

Bartlett and Burton (2006) describe the experience of a group of primary school teachers from nine schools in a networked learning community who wanted to inquire into their classroom teaching. Each teacher identified an educational intervention that they were developing in their classroom and that wanted to evaluate and decided what evidence was required and how to collect it. They frequently met with each other and with a mentor to share experiences and to discuss their work's progress. At the conclusion of their projects, they shared findings and their analysis with each other, with other teachers at their school and with teachers at other schools within the cluster. This is a typical example of a 'teacher-as-researcher' project. The authors suggest that the investigations be carried out by these teachers while counting as research also made significant contribution to their professional development.

Thus research in action research may be seen as the 'lubricant' to social action. As an outcome of the research, different forms of knowledge may be produced, 'practical knowledge' that can be used to implement the intervention and 'prepositional knowledge' that can be used for the development of generalizable theories (Sandars et al. 2012).

Sandars et al. (2012) highlight the transformative potential of action research in medical education based on the critical reflection of the findings that is inherent to it. In a limited review of action research studies in medical education, they identified 15 studies, the majority being on development and implementation of educational interventions and curriculum development.

2.3 Learning Theories

The debate on how people learn dates back to the time of the Greek philosophers. Plato (427–347 BC) espoused *rationalism*, that is, knowledge and truth can be found within us and therefore can be discovered by self-reflection. Socrates (469–399 BC) developed a dialectic approach to discovering truth through conversations with fellow citizens. Plato's student Aristotle (384–322 BC), on the other hand, was a proponent of *empiricism* that knowledge and truth was to be found outside of ourselves, using our senses, thus laying the foundation for the inquiry-based method (Darling-Hammond et al. 2001). Over the centuries, Western philosophers like Descartes, Rousseau, Kant and Locke continued the debate between Platonian rationalism and empiricism.

In the nineteenth century, the focus shifted from philosophy to a scientific study of learning. Edward Thorndike (1874–1949) first proposed a *behaviourist* theory of learning and described *connectionism* as a fundamental way of learning, that is, 'by the formation of associations between sensory experiences (stimuli) and neural impulses (responses) which manifest behaviorally' (Schunk 2012,). Influenced by Pavlov's experiments on classic conditioning, B. F. Skinner (1904–1990) proposed the operant conditioning theory comprising of the basic processes of reinforcement (positive or negative), punishment and the Premack principle that states 'the opportunity to engage in a more valued activity reinforces engaging in a less valued activity'. Behavioural change is brought about by *shaping* and *chaining*. Shaping refers to learning by doing with corrective feedback, where the learner is taken from initial to desired behaviour in small steps with constant reinforcement. Chaining is the process that influences skill learning, which involves several responses (steps) each of which alters the environment which in turn is the stimulus for the subsequent response.

Instructional applications of behavioural learning principles include the following:

1. Behaviour modification is a strategy that employs the principles of behavioural learning in diverse conditions including the classroom, for example, using shaping to address a specific annoying habit of a student.
2. Behavioural objectives are statements that clearly lay down intended outcomes of instruction and are useful in drawing up lesson plans and designing assessments of learning.
3. Mastery learning—although it contains cognitive elements, formulation of mastery learning seems to be more behavioural in nature (Schunk 2012). Mastery learning is based on the principle that if students are given the instruction that matches their individual aptitude, all students will demonstrate equal achievement. It includes the use of small group discussion formative assessments, individual tutorials and supplementary material. The mastery learning concept is applicable in the present-day recognition of the need for competency-based medical education (McGaghie 2015).
4. Programmed instruction refers to instructional material developed according to operant conditioning principles. An example is computer-based instruction where the learning objectives are provided to the student, the unit is divided into sequenced frames providing information incrementally, feedback is provided after each response and above all the learner proceeds at her own pace.

The conditioning theories were challenged in the 1950s and 1960s. Bandura's studies on observational learning demonstrated that learning can occur by observation without the need for reinforcement. His social cognitive theory is based on the idea that 'much human learning occurs in a social environment by observing others' (models). The theory also extends to include the role of self-regulation of behaviour. The social cognitive theory underscores a triadic reciprocality between persons, behaviour and the environment with a perceived self-efficacy influencing the choice of task, effort and skill acquisition. Modelling, using worked examples, tutoring and mentoring are some of the applications of the social cognitive theory (Schunk 2012).

Information processing, a key model in cognitive psychology, deals with sequence and execution of cognitive events (Schunk 2012). Information processing includes the processes of memory, attention and perception. Three types of memory are described—*sensory memory*, the first step in perception, from which information is passed to the *working memory* (WM) when the learner pays attention to it (Khalil and Elkhider 2016). From the working memory, information reaches the *long-term memory* (LTM) where it is stored in an encoded form and retrieved when needed. The WM is of limited capacity and duration, and for units to be retained in WM, rehearsal (repetition) is required (Schunk 2012). WM is useful when incoming information must be related to knowledge in LTM. In contrast, LTM has an unlimited capacity, and information is stored permanently and activated when cued. Information is encoded before it is stored in LTM. This occurs when new information is meaningful and can be integrated with known information in LTM. Encoding occurs by a process of *organization* of information into meaningful groups (chunking), by *elaboration* by which the new information is expanded upon and linked to what one already knows and by formation of *schemas* which have been described as 'cognitive constructs that incorporate multiple elements of information into a single element with a specific function' (Paas et al. 2003). Information is stored in LTM as propositions, and retrieval occurs by activating these propositional networks.

Instructional applications of information processing theories include:

1. Advance organizers—these are used at the beginning of a lesson to help connect new ideas with previous knowledge thereby setting the stage for meaningful learning. Organizers are derived from Ausubel's concept of 'meaningful learning' based on which he advocates *deductive teaching* (Schunk 2012). That is, general ideas are taught before going into specifics. Students break down ideas into smaller, related points and try to make links between new ideas and similar content in memory (expansion of propositional networks). Both these processes could be facilitated by the teacher.
2. Conditions of learning—described by Gagné, this refers to the circumstances that prevail when learning occurs and comprises a set of five learning outcomes and nine phases of learning. Gagné's conditions of learning have formed the basis of an instructional design model that has been explored for teaching psychomotor and procedural skills in medical education (Buscombe. 2013; Cheung 2016; Khadjooi et al. 2011).
3. Cognitive load—another well-known theory that has a widespread influence on instructional design is the cognitive load theory (CLT). This takes into account the limited capacity of the information processing function. Three types of cognitive load are described—*intrinsic* load that refers to the intrinsic properties of the information to be learnt and cannot be altered by instructional manipulation. Using simpler tasks can reduce this load, but eventually formation of an effective cognitive schema in LTM has to occur for understanding complex information (Paas et al. 2003). The second type of cognitive load is termed the *extraneous*

load which refers to the way in which information is presented to learners. Complex information (high intrinsic load) is better learnt when extraneous load is reduced so that the total cognitive load is within the processing capacity of the WM. The third type is termed *germane* load which indicates the learner's level of concentration devoted to learning, in other words, 'the load imposed by the mental processes necessary for learning (such as schemata formation and automation) to occur' (Young et al. 2014). One implication of the CLT is the reduction of extraneous load by scaffolding (simple to complex sequencing) (van Merrienboer et al. 2003) so that existing resources can be utilized for the intrinsic demands of learning. Other techniques to reduce the extraneous load include the use of goal-free tasks (Sweller et al. 1998), worked examples (Renkl and Atkinson 2003), use of authentic tasks in instruction and collaborative learning (Tolsgaard et al. 2016). Intrinsic load can be managed by moving from simple to complex tasks and low- to high-fidelity environment (van Merriënboer and Sweller 2010). Germane load can be optimized by encouraging cognitive strategies that facilitate schema construction, for example, introducing variability that mimic real-world situations into tasks (variability principle).

With an increasing focus on learners, educators have begun to question some of the assumptions of cognitive theories as they 'fail to capture the complexity of human learning' (Schunk 2012). Rather than as a theory, Hyslop-Margison and Strobel (2007) view constructivism as an epistemology (a philosophical explanation of the nature of learning). The central idea of constructivism is that knowledge is built within an individual and the interaction of persons and situations plays a key role in the acquisition of skills and knowledge (Cobb and Bowers 1999). In other words, cognitive processes are influenced by interactions between persons and the situation (situated cognition). Situated cognition is related to motivation, which is significantly influenced by the interaction of a learner's cognitive activities with sociocultural and instructional factors. Therefore, the appropriate instructional strategy is determined not just by the learning outcome but would vary with the individual student and the context in which learning is occurring (Hyslop-Margison and Strobel 2007).

Jean Piaget (1896–1980) proposed a theory of cognitive development that describes four discrete stages of development of an individual from birth to adulthood—sensorimotor (birth to 2 years), preoperational (2–7 years), concrete operational (7–11 years) and formal operational (11 to adult). He lists four factors that determine cognitive development, namely, the biological maturation of the individual, her experiences with the physical and social environment and equilibration. Equilibration is defined as a biological drive in an individual to produce an 'optimal state of equilibrium between cognitive structures and the environment' and occurs when a cognitive conflict exists, that is, when a mismatch is perceived between a learner's beliefs and observed reality (Schunk 2012). Piaget's theory implies the need for teachers to understand cognitive development to improve their teaching strategy, encourages the creation of incongruity and highlights the need for social interaction.

Vygotsky (1930–1934) proposed *social constructivism* as a theory of knowledge acquisition (Vygotsky 1978). It stresses the interactions between interpersonal cultural-historical and individual factors which cause learners to transform their experiences and reorganize their mental structures (Schunk 2012). Thus 'knowledge is a cultural and negotiated artifact generated in cooperation and understanding with others' (Hyslop-Margison and Strobel 2007). A key concept in Vygotsky's theory is the *zone of proximal development*, which refers to the difference between what a learner can do independently and what he can achieve under guidance or collaboration. Thus the instructor is a pivotal figure in the classroom who guides learners towards mastery with appropriate activities.

Instructional applications of Vygotsky's theory include:

1. Scaffolding—originally described by Wood, Bruner and Ross, this concept describes the use of various instructional tools to support student learning in the classroom, similar to Vygotsky's ZPD (Bentall and Allan 2014).
2. Reciprocal teaching—where the teacher and a small group of students are involved in an interactive dialogue with the students taking turns being the teacher.
3. Peer collaboration—which is also termed peer-assisted learning. In this instructional approach, peers are active agents in the learning process. Both tutors and tutees benefit from such programmes that need to be structured and monitored for efficacy. Peer tutoring has received much attention in both undergraduate and postgraduate medical education in recent years (Burgess et al. 2014; Hermann-Werner et al. 2017; Ten Cate and Durning 2007).
4. Apprenticeships—here novices learn from experts by working closely with experts in various work-related activities (Schunk 2012).

Dewey (1859–1952), in his model of constructivist learning, espoused the idea of 'constructing personal knowledge through individual cognition'. Focusing less on the sociocultural aspects of learner environment, it stresses on the creation of learning conditions that permit learners to pursue independent objectives based on their own experiences, interests and concerns (Hyslop-Margison and Strobel 2007). Thus the teacher is situated as a facilitator to help learners who are empowered to design their own learning experiences in accordance with their objectives and priorities.

2.4 The Research Scene in Medical Education

Medical education research (MER) took its roots in the United States in the 1950s with George Miller establishing the Office of Medical Education at the State University of New York, at Buffalo, New York (Norman 2011). Growth in scientific research in general, availability of funding, changes in accreditation policy that encouraged experimentation in medical education and increasing accountability of medical education were some factors that led to the establishment of MER at the time (Kuper et al. 2010). Since then scholarship in medical education has seen a steady rise in scope and intensity. Norman (2002) describes three generations of medical education researchers. The first generation consisted of faculty from backgrounds as varied as physics and economics. The second generation, established in the 1990s, comprised of medical education researchers from fields more closely related to education, namely, cognitive psychology and sociology and epidemiology, while the present generation of researchers hold degrees and doctorates in the field of medical education.

There has also been an exponential increase in the numbers of journals devoted to the publication of medical education research, Academic Medicine, Advances in Health Sciences Education, Medical Education, Medical Teacher and Teaching and Learning in Medicine, to name a few. Besides these journals that are solely devoted to the field of medical education research, some discipline-specific publications, such as the *Journal of American Medical Association*, *British Medical Journal* and *American Journal of Surgery*, have sections earmarked for publication of medical educational research papers. In a longitudinal review of MER publications in five major journals over 50 years, Lee et al. (2013) noted an increase in the number of Medline-indexed publications from 279 in 1960 to 3760 in 2010. There were more journals publishing medical education articles, 104 in 1960 to 855 in 2010. Also an increasing proportion of publications were of MER.

Research in medical education serves several purposes. It deepens knowledge and understanding of learning and education through the study of phenomena and 'how and why what works for whom' (Ringsted et al. 2011). It is also an opportunity for faculty who take a scholarly interest in the field and wish to publish for career advancement; it attempts to justify the time and resources spent on medical education activities and suggests a scientific approach to innovation. Curriculum and teaching issues including the use of technology, integration, the use of simulation and curricular evaluation are recurring themes for research (Regehr 2004). Other topics of interest include assessments, particularly emphasizing on authentic performance-based assessments such as workplace-based assessments (WPBA); student characteristics, including learning styles and motivation; admission policies on equity diversity and access; and studies on skills and attitudes, particularly on professionalism training and assessment.

Assessment has dominated the interest of medical education research over several decades. In a review of changing trends over two decades (1988–2010) from six of the major medical education publications, Rotgans (2012) noted that 26% of the research published was on issues of assessment. Reliability and validity of measures were found to be a recurring concern, and attention had shifted away from written (including MCQs) and oral forms of assessments to performance assessments. Assessments of the individual learner continue to be a major area of concern with the current move towards competency-based medical education (CBME) in which the design and implementation of assessments of competence pose a major challenge (Hamstra et al. 2014).

Rotgans identified 28 other themes for research including clinical skill training, clinical clerkships and problem-based learning (PBL). A few newer themes have emerged such as issues of patient safety, humanities in medicine and interprofessional education. Research in preclinical education has also seen an increase with journals such as *Anatomical Sciences Education* and Advances in Physiological Education being established by the professional bodies in these disciplines (Annotated Bibliography of Journals for Educational Scholarship Revised March 2016).

Hamstra (2012) identifies seven major thrust areas for research in the future, including:

1. Contextual issues such as philosophical foundations of medicine and medical education and sociocultural issues in clinical teaching.
2. Cognition and educational theory.
3. Individual assessment including WPBA and assessment of noncognitive skills.
4. Teaching and learning issues, namely, effective teaching of clinical skills, community orientation and training for continuity of care.
5. Curriculum development, design and evaluation.
6. Leadership development.
7. Methodology and research principles.

Research in medical education is now an established field (Norman 2002). Significant evidence has accumulated in several areas such as basic research on the acquisition of expertise, PBL, assessment and continuing education. Rotgans (2012) identifies five major innovations from medical education research since the 1960s. These include problem-based learning (PBL), objective structured clinical examination (OSCE), the description of a systematic approach to training of professional skills and establishing that clinical reasoning is to a large extent knowledge based and that global ratings are more valid than checklists.

MER includes a wide range of study designs and methods encompassing both quantitative and qualitative approaches. Ringsted et al. (2011) propose a conceptual model for the underlying theoretic framework to medical education research. They describe four categories of studies, namely, explorative, experimental, observational and translational. Explorative studies are characterized by the exploration of phenomena and employ a predominantly qualitative approach.

Experimental studies propose to establish evidence of the effects of an intervention. By carefully controlling the conditions of the experiment, the researcher tries to minimize the effects of confounders. There are many types of experimental studies. The classical randomized controlled trial (RCT) design that is employed in biomedical research is also used in educational research. It is worth noting that the RCT which is considered the highest in the hierarchy of levels of evidence in biomedical research may not be the ideal for much of education research. Though there are many who argue vehemently for its value (Cook 2002; Goldacre 2013; Todres et al. 2007), there are those who equally vehemently question its importance in education research (Norman 2003; Sullivan 2011). Other experimental designs described in medical education research include the Solomon four-group RCT design, the randomized post-test-only design, the single-group pre- and post-design, the single-group post-test-only design and the no intervention comparison study design.

The third category of educational studies in Ringsted's 'research compass' (Ringsted et al. 2011) includes observational studies, such as cohort, case control and association studies that seek to predict outcomes. The challenge to observational studies is that they can't be controlled for bias and it is difficult to establish causal relationships. They can thus serve as precursors to experimental studies.

The final category includes translational studies that include investigations into the processes of transfer of basic educational science into everyday medical education practices and those that study how learning in the classroom translates into practice in real life. They include knowledge creation studies such as systematic reviews, knowledge implementation studies and efficiency studies that investigate complex interventions.

Medical education research faces several challenges (Shea et al. 2004; Gruppen 2007):

1. In the practical setting of teaching and student affairs, research is usually not a priority.
2. Conflicting demands on time for clinicians with lack of protected time for MER.
3. Researchers themselves may face the tension between the demand for more practical research from 'consumers' (production for users) and the need for conducting theory-based research for the advancement of the field (production for producers) (Albert et al. 2007).
4. It occurs in a constantly evolving context that does not give sufficient time to plan a good study, for example, students are exposed to different curricula at any given time, and intervention in one curriculum may be affected by concurrent curricula, making interpretation difficult.
5. What works in one setting may not work in another.
6. The diversity among researchers who have varying levels of training and experience in MER may result in varying standards and perspectives for research.
7. Lack of funding is a significant barrier to high-quality educational research (Davis 2006).

These challenges may be overcome by training of researchers in research methods (Gruppen 2007), providing adequate funding and technical support for better research, encouraging collaboration between researchers (producers) and clinicians (users) and opening up MER to researchers from other fields such as the social sciences (Albert et al. 2007).

2.5 Bridging the Research-Practice Gap: Appraising the Research and Using the Evidence

Two main outcomes obtained from educational research include understanding and building the theory of learning and assessment and implementing innovative solutions to problems in the field. It is also believed that uptake and application of research evidence to improve educational practices will ultimately result in improved patient care, what is termed as knowledge translation (Thomas and Bussières 2016a, b). Knowledge that is based on and substantiated by research can be utilized in a material form such as a protocol or a set of guidelines (instrumental utilization), to change one's way of thinking that may not necessarily be accompanied by behavioural change (conceptual utilization) or 'as a persuasive tool to legitimize a position or practice', such as accreditation standards (persuasive/symbolic utilization).

It is generally perceived that there exists a research-practice gap (Cook et al. 2008; MacLellan 2016; van der Vleuten and Driessen 2014). Foremost among the reasons for this is the researcher-practitioner gap and the weak communication that exists between the two groups of professionals. Contributors to this undesirable situation include difficulty in understanding the language of educational research (use of jargon), inaccessibility of the literature (most of the publications are in journals dedicated to educational research that may not be available in school libraries), large volume and lack of time to read the published literature, feeling that the research is irrelevant, too theoretical and unhelpful to the practitioner (Hemsley-Brown and Sharp 2003) and a perception among users that the research is done more as an academic study than to support their teaching. A similar situation exists in the use of research evidence in medical practice too (Hemsley-Brown and Sharp 2003). Making the information more easily available and accessible, enabling teachers to have time to read the research, providing evidence of benefits, ensuring that research has practical application, involving practitioners at all steps of the project (although there is a possibility that the resistance from only the group of practitioners directly involved would be overcome) and identifying change agents who would 'translate' the research findings for users and opinion leaders with the required credibility within peer networks to 'diffuse' the innovation to others are some strategies that can facilitate use of research by practitioners.

Implementation science is the scientific study of knowledge translation. Thomas and Bussières (2016a, b) describe it as four-step process that uses scientific evidence underpinned by theories, frameworks and models to achieve knowledge translation. The four steps include identifying research-practice gaps, identifying barriers and supports to uptake of research evidence, designing interventions to reduce the research-practice gaps and evaluating the impact of interventions on educational practice (Thomas and Bussières 2016a, b).

Several criticisms have been levelled at medical education research. Lack of rigour is an oft-cited shortcoming. Small sample sizes with often lack of a comparison group, issues of randomization, errors in measurement, inappropriate statistical tools, poor standards for reporting results making it difficult to interpret results and to replicate the study and using low-level outcome measures that focus mostly on learner reactions and assessment scores rather than on more rigorous outcomes such as physician behaviours are some commonly observed deficiencies (Gruppen 2007; Picho and Artino 2016). Poor research questions, inadequate detail in the description of methods and context, too small or biased samples, inappropriate or insufficiently described statistics, insufficient data being presented and paucity of literature review are some of the issues identified as reasons for rejecting manuscripts submitted for publication (Bordage 2001). Medical education research is seen to be more an effectiveness-driven than discovery-driven exercise, that is, the results of research focus more on effectiveness of existing approaches rather than on discovering new ones (Regehr 2004).

In addition, gaps in researchers' theoretical knowledge and in their training in research methodology particularly in methods used in social sciences research have been cited as having a negative impact on the quality of research in medical education (Albert et al. 2007).

Cook et al. (2008) note that 'many research studies in medical education fail to follow a line of inquiry that over time will advance the science in the field' and proposes a framework for classifying the purpose of medical education research. They suggest three categories that studies could be grouped into:

1. Description studies that are based on observation and involve no comparisons, for example, a report on a new assessment method.
2. Justification studies that involve comparison of educational interventions to answer the question 'Does the new intervention work?' These usually involve the use of RCT.
3. Clarification studies that address the questions 'How does it work?' and 'Why does it work?' They usually begin with observations and models or theories on the basis of which predictions are made which are then tested. A range of study designs can be used for such studies that are characterized by 'the presence of a conceptual framework or theory that can be affirmed or refuted by the results of the study'.

In an analysis of 110 papers on experimental studies published in 2003 and 2004 in 4 leading medical education journals, Cook (2008) found that 72% of the papers fell into the justification category, 13% into the description category and 12% into the clarification group.

When appraising the evidence obtained from health professions education research, the following criteria of quality are considered with respect to quantitative studies—*trustworthiness*, that is, the truth of the evidence; *generalizability* of evidence or, in other words, its applicability in other settings; *consistency* of the evidence, that is, results are consistent when the study is replicated; and *neutrality* of evidence, referring to the absence of biases (Frambach et al. 2013).

Trustworthiness of the evidence from a study reflects its internal validity. A study's internal validity refers to the extent to which observed effects can be attributed to the independent variable, that is, whether inferences can be drawn about a causal relationship between two variables. Some threats to internal validity include *history*, referring to events that may be occurring concurrently with the treatment and which may be responsible for the observed effect; *maturation*, referring to changes that are naturally occurring over time and which may be misinterpreted as treatment effect; *attrition*, loss of respondents to the treatment; *testing effect*, whereby a prior exposure to a test can affect scores on subsequent exposure to the test; and *instrumentation*, referring to changes that may be made to the measuring instrument over time (e.g. changing the items in a test as the study progresses) in ways that may influence the results leading to confusion in interpretation (Torre and

Picho 2016). The internal validity of a study can be enhanced by applying a 'power calculation' for the sample size, using a controlled design, standardizing the treatment conditions, avoiding loss of participants or providing information on non-responses and describing the educational context and the intervention in detail (Frambach et al. 2013).

External validity of a study may be defined as 'the extent to which the conclusions of the study would hold for variations in persons, treatment and outcomes'. The more these vary from those of a given study, the less generalizable its findings. Thus, factors that reduce the generalizability of a study include employing a sample that is homogenous or in some way unusual, conducting the study in an atypical setting, using an atypical treatment, listing inappropriate outcomes or conducting the study at a peculiar time in history. External validity can be increased by random sampling, selecting multiple sites and replicating the study with different people in a variety of settings with different sets of dependent and independent variables (Artino et al. 2011).

It is worthwhile noting that external and internal validity are often in conflict in a particular study. Conditions that increase internal validity, for example, a study that is being done under tightly controlled conditions, may result in a decrease in its generalizability and vice versa.

The reliability of a study that refers to the extent to which the results of a study are obtained consistently when the study is replicated can be increased by estimating the internal consistency across repeated measures and the sources of variance affecting the measurement. Objectivity of the study that ensures neutrality of the evidence can be enhanced by maintaining anonymity of respondent identities, blinding the assessors of the data and preserving the original data for accountability to public and publishers (Frambach 2013).

When appraising or designing qualitative studies, the Total Quality Framework (Roller and Lavrakas 2015) is a useful set of criteria to employ. The framework describes four major criteria, namely credibility, analysability, transparency and usefulness.

Credibility includes the scope of the study and its construct validity that is reflected by the data-gathering process. The scope refers to 'all those aspects of the study that affect the extent to which the final sample from (or about) which data are gathered reflects the important characteristics of the target population that is being studied'. The construct validity is determined by 'how well the data gathered actually represents what the researchers claim to measure'.

Analysability is dependent on the credibility component and refers to the need to process and analyse data completely and accurately to produce valid and useful findings. It includes the processing of the data to enable analysis such as transcribing recorded interviews and the data analysis itself to develop codes, themes and categories.

Transparency is concerned with the disclosure of all aspects related to the credibility and analysability of a qualitative study in the final documentation. This is achieved using 'thick descriptions' that include rich details which will allow the reader to better determine its applicability.

Usefulness refers to the use of the study not only to the researchers themselves but also to other users of the research.

Harden et al. (1999) suggest a multidimensional approach to grading evidence. The six dimensions each with its own continuum refer to quality, utility, extent, strength, target and setting of the evidence and are represented by the acronym QUESTS.

Quality of evidence from a research study is judged by posing relevant questions regarding the background of the study, the sample, data collection process, data analysis, the validity, reliability and generalizability of the findings and the conclusions and recommendations that follow from it. If the evidence is based on theory, opinion or experience, questions would address the acceptability of the approach, the level of expertise of the practitioner and whether the view expressed is of relevance to medical education and its values.

Utility refers to 'the extent to which the method or intervention described in the original report can be transplanted to another situation without adaptation'.

The extent of evidence denotes the number of studies that the evidence is based on, whether a single study, a consensus view, a systematic review or a meta-analysis of a number of studies.

Strength of evidence is reflected in the statistical significance of the results.

The target for the evidence refers to the outcomes that have been measured, that is, the research question that has been asked. The authors list this dimension as the most important one when evaluating evidence as it is related to the validity or practical relevance of the findings. They describe a modified version of Kirkpatrick's levels with impact as the highest level, for instance, on health outcomes of the population. However, evaluating evidence in terms of such impact is not always feasible and is made more difficult by the number of confounding factors. Yardley and Dornan (2012) argue that viewing Kirkpatrick's various levels as a hierarchy may not be applicable, as in some situations, a level 1 evidence (participant reactions) is important for policy making, curriculum designing and when assessing students' experiences.

The last dimension of the QUESTS approach to evaluating evidence refers to the setting or context in which it is gathered. This is important with respect to transferability of the findings, as 'teaching practice is context and culturally specific, and research findings in one area may be of limited value to those in different practice settings' (Harden et al. 1999).

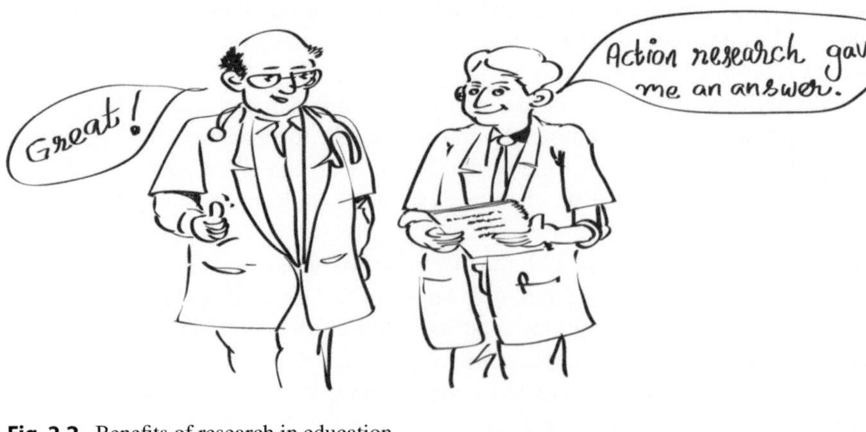

Fig. 2.2 Benefits of research in education

Conclusions

Evidence from educational research is highly contextual. What is shown to work well with one set of learners may not necessarily apply with learners from a different situation.

Research, particularly teacher-conducted research, contributes to curriculum improvement by providing an opportunity to understand and test the applicability of the theoretical principles in education and thus a rational basis for bringing in desired changes in the curriculum.

References

Adelman C (1993) Kurt Lewin and the origins of action research. Educ Action Res 1:7–24. https://doi.org/10.1080/0965079930010102

Albert M, Hodges B, Regehr G (2007) Research in medical education: balancing service and science. Adv Health Sci Educ 12:103–115. https://doi.org/10.1007/s10459-006-9026-2

Annotated Bibliography of Journals for Educational Scholarship; Revised March 2016. Accessed online from https://www.aamc.org/download/184694/data/annotated_bibliography_of_journals.pdf

Anshu, Grant J (2014) Mixed methods research and evaluation. FAIMER-Keele Master's in Health Professions Education: accreditation and assessment. Module 4, Unit 1. FAIMER Centre for Distance Learning, CenMEDIC, London

Artino AR, Durning SJ, Boulet JR (2011) Generalizability in medical education research. Acad Med 86(7):917

Barnett-Page E, Thomas J (2009) Methods for the synthesis of qualitative research: a critical review. BMC Med Res Methodol 9. https://doi.org/10.1186/1471-2288-9-59

Bartlett S, Burton D (2006) Practitioner research or descriptions of classroom practice? A discussion of teachers investigating their classrooms. Educ Action Res 14:395–405. https://doi.org/10.1080/09650790600847735

Bentall C, Allan H (2014) Learning theories. A critique. FAIMER-Keele Master's in Health Professions Education: accreditation and assessment. Module 6, Unit 1. FAIMER Centre for Distance Learning, CenMEDIC, London

Biesta G (2007) Bridging the gap between educational research and educational practice: the need for critical distance. Educ Res Eval 13:295–301. https://doi.org/10.1080/13803610701640227

Bordage G (2001) Reasons reviewers reject and accept manuscripts: the strengths and weaknesses in medical education reports. Acad Med 76:889–896

Brannen (2005) Accessed online from http://eprints.ncrm.ac.uk/89/1/MethodsReviewPaperNCRM-005.pdf

Bunniss S, Kelly DR (2010) Research paradigms in medical education research. Med Educ 44:358–366. https://doi.org/10.1111/j.1365-2923.2009.03611.x

Burgess A, McGregor D, Mellis C (2014) Medical students as peer tutors: a systematic review. BMC Med Educ 14:115

Buscombe C (2013) Using Gagne's theory to teach procedural skills. Clin Teach 10:302–307

Chen HC, Teherani A (2016) A common qualitative methodologies and research designs in health professions education. Acad Med 91(12):e5

Cheung L (2016) Using an instructional design model to teach medical procedures. Med Sci Educ 26:175–180. https://doi.org/10.1007/s40670-016-0228-9

Clegg S (2005) Evidence-based practice in educational research: a critical realist critique of systematic review. Br J Sociol Educ 26:415–428. https://doi.org/10.1080/01425690500128932

Cleland J, Jamieson S (2014) Quantitative research methods. FAIMER-Keele Master's in Health Professions Education: accreditation and assessment. Module 4, Unit 4. FAIMER Centre for Distance Learning, CenMEDIC, London

Cobb P, Bowers J (1999) Cognitive and situated learning perspectives in theory and practice. Educ Res 28:4–15. https://doi.org/10.3102/0013189X028002004

Cook TD (2002) Randomized experiments in educational policy research: a critical examination of the reasons the educational evaluation community has offered for not doing them. Educ Eval Policy Anal 24:175–199

Cook DA (2008) Narrowing the focus and broadening horizons: complementary roles for systematic and nonsystematic reviews. Adv Health Sci Educ 13:391–395. https://doi.org/10.1007/s10459-008-9140-4

Cook DA, Bordage G, Schmidt HG (2008) Description, justification and clarification: a framework for classifying the purposes of research in medical education: description, justification and clarification. Med Educ 42:128–133. https://doi.org/10.1111/j.1365-2923.2007.02974.x

Darling-Hammond L, Austin K, Orcutt S, Rosso J (2001) "How people learn: introduction to learning theories", The learning classroom: theory into practice. A telecourse for teacher education and professional development. Stanford University School of Education, Stanford, CA, Episode1

Davies P (1999) What is evidence-based education? Br J Educ Stud 47:108–121. https://doi.org/10.1111/1467-8527.00106

Davis MH, Ponnamperuma GG (2006) Medical education research at the crossroads. The Lancet 367(9508):377–378

van der Vleuten CPM, Driessen EW (2014) What would happen to education if we take education evidence seriously? Perspect Med Educ 3:222–232. https://doi.org/10.1007/s40037-014-0129-9

Dixon-Woods M, Agarwal S, Jones D, Young B, Sutton A (2005) Synthesising qualitative and quantitative evidence: a review of possible methods. J Health Serv Res Policy 10:45–53. https://doi.org/10.1258/1355819052801804

Dixon-Woods M, Cavers D, Agarwal S, Annandale E, Arthur A, Harvey J, Hsu R, Katbamna S, Olsen R, Smith L, Riley R, Sutton AJ (2006) Conducting a critical interpretive synthesis of the literature on access to healthcare by vulnerable groups. BMC Med Res Methodol 6. https://doi.org/10.1186/1471-2288-6-35

Eva KW (2008) On the limits of systematicity. Med Educ 42:852–853. https://doi.org/10.1111/j.1365-2923.2008.03140.x

Fraenkel JR, Wallen NE, Hyun HH (2011) How to design and evaluate research in education, 8th edn. McGraw-Hill Humanities/Social Sciences/Languages, New York

Frambach JM, van der Vleuten CPM, Durning SJ (2013) Quality criteria in qualitative and quantitative research. Acad Med 88(4):552

Glassman M, Erdem G, Bartholomew M (2013) Action research and its history as an adult education movement for social change. Adult Educ Q 63:272–288

Goldacre B, Department for Education (DFE), corp creator (2013) Building evidence into education. [Bad science]. Available from http://dera.ioe.ac.uk/17530/

Gordon M, Patricio MF (2016) Best evidence medical and health professional education (BEME) collaboration: a moving spotlight. Med Teach 38:1–2. https://doi.org/10.3109/0142159X.2015.1074991

Greenhalgh T, Robert G, Macfarlane F, Bate P, Kyriakidou O, Peacock R (2005) Storylines of research in diffusion of innovation: a meta-narrative approach to systematic review. Soc Sci Med 61:417–430. https://doi.org/10.1016/j.socscimed.2004.12.001

Gruppen LD (2007) Improving medical education research. Teach Learn Med 19:331–335. https://doi.org/10.1080/10401330701542370

Hammersley M (2012) Methodological paradigms in educational research, British Educational Research Association online resource. Available online at https://www.bera.ac.uk/researchers-resources/publications/methodological-paradigms-in-educational-research

Hamstra SJ (2012) Keynote address: the focus on competencies and individual learner assessment as emerging themes in medical education research. Acad Emerg Med 19:1336–1343. https://doi.org/10.1111/acem.12021

Hamstra S, Schoenherr J, Falconer M (2014) Emerging themes in medical education research. Clin Med Educ 1:6–11

Harden M, Grant J, Buck GR (1999) BEME Guide No. 1: best evidence medical education. Med Teach 21:553–562. https://doi.org/10.1080/01421599978960
Hathaway RS (1995) Assumptions underlying quantitative and qualitative research: implications for institutional research. Res High Educ 36:535–562
Hemsley-Brown J, Sharp C (2003) The use of research to improve professional practice: a systematic review of the literature. Oxf Rev Educ 29:449–471. https://doi.org/10.1080/0305498032000153025
Herrmann-Werner A, Gramer R, Erschens R, Nikendei C, Wosnik A, Griewatz J, Zipfel S, Junne F (2017) Peer-assisted learning (PAL) in undergraduate medical education: an overview. Z Evid Fortbild Qual Gesundhwes 121:74–81. https://doi.org/10.1016/j.zefq.2017.01.001
Hyslop-Margison EJ, Strobel J (2007) Constructivism and education: misunderstandings and pedagogical implications. Teach Educ 43:72–86. https://doi.org/10.1080/08878730701728945
Khadjooi K, Rostami K, Ishaq S (2011) How to use Gagne's model of instructional design in teaching psychomotor skills. Gastroenterol Hepatol Bed Bench 4:116
Khalil MK, Elkhider IA (2016) Applying learning theories and instructional design models for effective instruction. Adv Physiol Educ 40:147–156. https://doi.org/10.1152/advan.00138.2015
Kuper A, Lingard L, Levinson W (2008) Critically appraising qualitative research. BMJ 337:a1035–a1035. https://doi.org/10.1136/bmj.a1035
Kuper A, Albert M, Hodges BD (2010) The origins of the field of medical education research. Acad Med 85:1347–1353. https://doi.org/10.1097/ACM.0b013e3181dce9a7
Lee K, Whelan JS, Tannery NH, Kanter SL, Peters AS (2013) 50 years of publication in the field of medical education. Med Teach 35:591–598. https://doi.org/10.3109/0142159X.2013.786168
Lemons CJ, Fuchs D, Gilbert JK, Fuchs LS (2014) Evidence-based practices in a changing world: reconsidering the counterfactual in education research. Educ Res 43:242–252
Levinson AJ (2010) Where is evidence-based instructional design in medical education curriculum development?: commentaries. Med Educ 44:536–537. https://doi.org/10.1111/j.1365-2923.2010.03715.x
Lucas PJ, Baird J, Arai L, Law C, Roberts HM (2007) Worked examples of alternative methods for the synthesis of qualitative and quantitative research in systematic reviews. BMC Med Res Methodol 7. https://doi.org/10.1186/1471-2288-7-4
Lukenchuk A, Kolich E (2013) Chapter 3: Paradigms and educational research: weaving the tapestry. Counterpoints 436:61–87 www.jstor.org/stable/42981910
MacLellan (2016) Why don't teachers use education research in teaching? Accessed online at https://eic.rsc.org/analysis/why-dont-teachers-use-education-research-in-teaching/2010170.article
MacLeod A (2016) Understanding the culture of graduate medical education: the benefits of ethnographic research. J Grad Med Educ 8:142–144. https://doi.org/10.4300/JGME-D-15-00069.1
MacLure M (2005) 'Clarity bordering on stupidity': where's the quality in systematic review? J Educ Policy 20:393–416. https://doi.org/10.1080/02680930500131801
Mayer RE (2010) Applying the science of learning to medical education: applying the science of learning. Med Educ 44:543–549. https://doi.org/10.1111/j.1365-2923.2010.03624.x
McGaghie WC (2015) Mastery learning: it is time for medical education to join the 21st century. Acad Med 90:1438–1441. https://doi.org/10.1097/ACM.0000000000000911
McTaggart R (1994) Participatory action research: issues in theory and practice. Educ Action Res 2(3):313–337. https://doi.org/10.1080/0965079940020302
van Merriënboer JJ, Sweller J (2010) Cognitive load theory in health professional education: design principles and strategies. Med Educ 44:85–93. https://doi.org/10.1111/j.1365-2923.2009.03498.x
van Merrienboer JJG, Kirschner PA, Kester L (2003) Taking the load off a learner's mind: instructional design for complex learning. Educ Psychol 38:5–13. https://doi.org/10.1207/S15326985EP3801_2
Norman G (2002) Research in medical education: three decades of progress. BMJ 324:1560–1562
Norman G (2003) RCT = results confounded and trivial: the perils of grand educational experiments. Med Educ 37:582–584

Norman G (2011) Fifty years of medical education research: waves of migration: history of medical education research. Med Educ 45:785–791. https://doi.org/10.1111/j.1365-2923.2010.03921.x
Paas F, Renkl A, Sweller J (2003) Cognitive load theory and instructional design: recent developments. Educ Psychol 38:1–4. https://doi.org/10.1207/S15326985EP3801_1
Patrício M, vaz Carneiro A (2012) Systematic reviews of evidence in medical education and clinical medicine: is the nature of evidence similar? Med Teach 34:474–482. https://doi.org/10.3109/0142159X.2012.682186
Picho K, Artino AR (2016) 7 deadly sins in educational research. J Grad Med Educ 8:483–487. https://doi.org/10.4300/JGME-D-16-00332.1
Reeves S, Peller J, Goldman J, Kitto S (2013) Ethnography in qualitative educational research: AMEE Guide No. 80. Med Teach 35:e1365–e1379. https://doi.org/10.3109/0142159X.2013.804977
Regehr G (2004) Trends in medical education research. Acad Med 79:939–947
Renkl A, Atkinson RK (2003) Structuring the transition from example study to problem solving in cognitive skill acquisition: a cognitive load perspective. Educ Psychol 38:15–22. https://doi.org/10.1207/S15326985EP3801_3
Ringsted C, Hodges B, Scherpbier A (2011) 'The research compass': an introduction to research in medical education: AMEE Guide No. 56. Med Teach 33:695–709. https://doi.org/10.3109/0142159X.2011.595436
Roller MR, Lavrakas PJ (2015) Applied qualitative research design a total quality framework approach. The Guilford Press, New York
Rotgans JI (2012) The themes, institutions, and people of medical education research 1988–2010: content analysis of abstracts from six journals. Adv Health Sci Educ 17:515–527. https://doi.org/10.1007/s10459-011-9328-x
Sackett DL, Rosenberg WMC, Gray JAM, Haynes RB, Richardson WS (1996) Evidence based medicine: what it is and what it isn't. BMJ 312:71–72. https://doi.org/10.1136/bmj.312.7023.71
Sandars J, Singh G, MacLeod S (2012) Are we missing the potential of action research for transformative change in medical education? Educ Prim Care 23:239–241. https://doi.org/10.1080/14739879.2012.11494115
Schunk DH (2012) Learning theories: an educational perspective, 6th edn. Pearson, Boston
Shea JA, Arnold L, Mann KV (2004) A RIME perspective on the quality and relevance of current and future medical education research. Acad Med 79:931–938
Stalmeijer RE, McNaughton N, Van Mook WNKA (2014) Using focus groups in medical education research: AMEE Guide No. 91. Med Teach 36:923–939. https://doi.org/10.3109/0142159X.2014.917165
Stenhouse L (1979) Research as a basis for teaching an inaugural lecture by Lawrence Stenhouse, University of East Anglia. Accessed online at https://www.uea.ac.uk/documents/4059364/4994243/Stenhouse-1979-Research+as+a+Basis+for+Teaching.pdf/8a005112-a420-4e39-85a0-0fde58d4846d
Stewart J, Filice de Barros N (2014) Qualitative research methods. FAIMER-Keele Master's in Health Professions Education: accreditation and assessment. Module 4, Unit 6. FAIMER Centre for Distance Learning, CenMEDIC, London, p 6
Sullivan GM (2011) Getting off the "gold standard": randomized controlled trials and education research. J Grad Med Educ 3:285–289. https://doi.org/10.4300/JGME-D-11-00147.1
Sweller J, Van Merrienboer JJ, Paas FG (1998) Cognitive architecture and instructional design. Educ Psychol Rev 10:251–296
Taylor PC, Medina MND (2013) Educational research paradigms: from positivism to multiparadigmatic. The Journal of Meaning-Centered Education 1:1–13
Ten Cate O, Durning S (2007) Peer teaching in medical education: twelve reasons to move from theory to practice. Med Teach 29:591–599. https://doi.org/10.1080/01421590701606799
Thistlethwaite J, Hammick M (2010) The Best Evidence Medical Education (BEME) collaboration: into the next decade. Med Teach 32:880–882. https://doi.org/10.3109/0142159X.2010.519068
Thistlethwaite J, Davies H, Dornan T, Greenhalgh T, Hammick M, Scalese R (2012) What is evidence? Reflections on the AMEE symposium, Vienna, Aug 2011. Med Teach 34:454–457. https://doi.org/10.3109/0142159X.2012.671561

Thomas A, Bussières A (2016a) Towards a greater understanding of implementation science in health professions education. Acad Med 91(12):e19. https://doi.org/10.1097/ACM.0000000000001441

Thomas A, Bussières A (2016b) A knowledge translation and implementation science in health professions education: time for clarity? Acad Med 91(12):e20. https://doi.org/10.1097/ACM.0000000000001396

Thomas J, Harden A (2008) Methods for the thematic synthesis of qualitative research in systematic reviews. BMC Med Res Methodol 8. https://doi.org/10.1186/1471-2288-8-45

Todres M, Stephenson A, Jones R (2007) Medical education research remains the poor relation. BMJ 335:333

Tolsgaard MG, Kulasegaram KM, Ringsted CV (2016) Collaborative learning of clinical skills in health professions education: the why, how, when and for whom. Med Educ 50:69–78. https://doi.org/10.1111/medu.12814

Torre DM, Picho K (2016) Threats to internal and external validity in health professions education research. Acad Med 91(12):e21

Tranfield D, Denyer D, Smart P (2003) Towards a methodology for developing evidence-informed management knowledge by means of systematic review. Br J Manag 14:207–222

Tripp D (2005) Action research: a methodological introduction. Educ Pesqui 31(3):443–466. https://doi.org/10.1590/S1517-97022005000300009

Van der Mescht H (2004) Phenomenology in education: a case study in educational leadership. Indo-Pacific Journal of Phenomenology 4:1–16. https://doi.org/10.1080/20797222.2004.11433887

Vygotsky LS (1978) In: Cole M, John-Steiner V, Scribner S, Souberman E (eds) Mind in society: the development of higher psychological processes (Luria AR, Lopez-Morillas M, Cole M [with J. V. Wertsch], trans.). Harvard University Press, Cambridge, MA (Original manuscripts [ca. 1930–1934])

Watling CJ, Lingard L (2012) Grounded theory in medical education research: AMEE Guide No. 70. Med Teach 34:850–861. https://doi.org/10.3109/0142159X.2012.704439

Yardley S, Dornan T (2012) Kirkpatrick's levels and education 'evidence': Kirkpatrick's levels in education. Med Educ 46:97–106. https://doi.org/10.1111/j.1365-2923.2011.04076.x

Young JQ, Van Merrienboer J, Durning S, Ten Cate O (2014) Cognitive load theory: implications for medical education: AMEE Guide No. 86. Med Teach 36:371–384. https://doi.org/10.3109/0142159X.2014.889290

Part III

Improving Discipline-based Undergraduate Medical Curriculum

Social Accountability

3

Objectives
1. Describe the rationale for social accountability of medical schools.
2. Define and describe important features of social accountability of medical schools.
3. Give some examples of the adoption of the concept of social accountability.
4. Describe the measures to improve social accountability of undergraduate medical education.

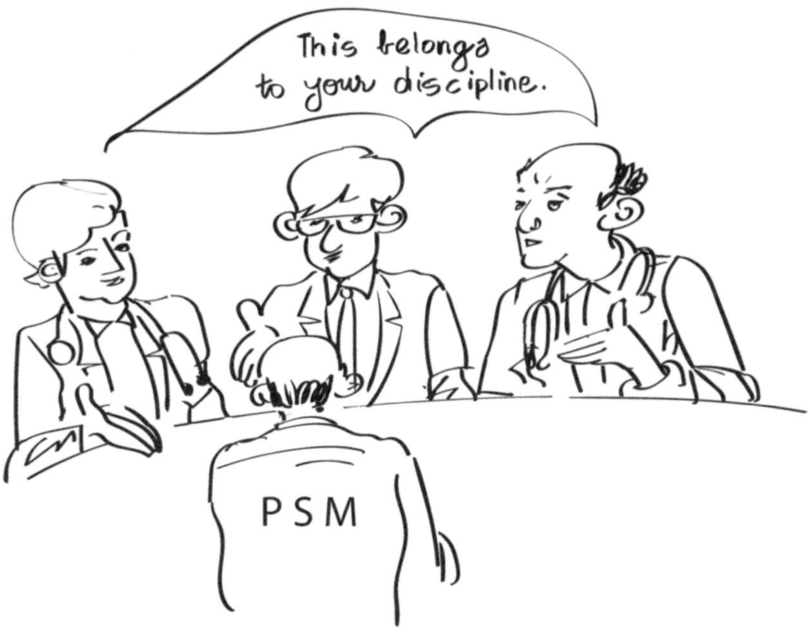

Fig. 3.1 Social accountability-isolated responsibility

Kadambari D et al., *Improving Discipline-Based Undergraduate Medical Curriculum*, https://doi.org/10.1007/978-981-13-1310-3_3

3.1 Introduction

The purpose of medical profession is to serve the health needs of society. In other words, medical profession has the responsibility of serving the societal health needs. Medical profession uses service, education and research for serving the societal health needs. Thus there is social responsibility of medical profession. As part of this, there is also social responsibility of medical schools. In 1995, the concept of social accountability of medical schools was introduced (Boelen and Heck 1995). Over the years, this concept has become widely accepted. The concept of social accountability has the advantage of including the evaluation of impact on health needs which makes it possible to ensure that societal health needs have been fulfilled.

3.2 Rationale for Social Accountability

3.2.1 Human Right to Health

Health is essential for optimal functioning of a human being. The World Health Organization (2006) in its constitution has defined health as given below.

> Health is a state of complete physical, mental and social well-being not merely the absence of disease or infirmity.

All human beings are entitled to certain rights. The constitution of the World Health Organization (2006) states that health is a human right as mentioned below.

> The enjoyment of the highest attainable standard of health is one of the fundamental rights of every human being without distinction of race, religion, political belief, economic or social condition.

The United Nations Universal Declaration of Human Rights in its Article 25 (United Nations 1948) includes the following.

> Everyone has the right to a standard of living adequate for the health and well-being of himself and of his family….

3.2.2 Health for All by the Year 2000

The World Health Organization launched the concept of Health for All by the Year 2000 and published *Global Strategy for Health for All by the Year 2000* (World Health Organization 1981). This was a logical progression of the acceptance of the idea that health is a fundamental human right.

During the period of Health for All by the Year 2000 programme, global, regional and national recommendations were made for aligning medical education to health-care needs of the society. The Edinburgh Declaration of World Conference on Medical Education (World Federation for Medical Education 1988) comprised 12 principles including the following:

> The basing of curricula on national health needs.

The goal of Reorientation of Medical Education programme for Southeast Asia (World Health Organization 1988) was:

> … that by the year 2000, all medical schools in the region will be producing, according to the needs and resources of the country, graduate or specialist doctors, who are responsive to the social and societal needs and who possess the appropriate ethical, social, technical and management abilities so as to enable them to work effectively in the comprehensive health system based on primary health care which are being developed in the countries of the Region.

National Health Policy (Government of India 1983) stated the following:

> It is, therefore, of crucial importance that the entire basis and approach towards medical and health education, at all levels, is reviewed in terms of national needs and priorities and curricular and training programmes restructured to produce personnel of various grades of skill and competence, who are professionally equipped and socially motivated to effectively deal with day-to-day problems within existing constraints.

In spite of global and national efforts, the progress towards Health for All by the Year 2000 was below expectations. This was one of the factors which led to the introduction of the concept of social accountability of medical schools in the year 1995.

3.3 Social Accountability of Medical Schools

3.3.1 Definition

Boelen and Heck (1995) first defined social accountability of medical schools, and the definition is currently recognized (Boelen et al. 2016) as:

> …the obligation of medical schools to direct their education, research and service activities towards addressing the priority health needs of the community, region, and/or nation they have a mandate to serve. The priority health needs are to be identified jointly by governments, health care organizations, health professionals and the public.

3.3.2 Four Values/Principles of Social Accountability

Four values/principles of quality, equity, relevance and effectiveness are essential to achieve social accountability (Boelen et al. 2012). These values are used for planning and implementing programmes. Definitions of these values/principles (Boelen et al. 2012) are cited below.

> Quality is the measure by which satisfactory responses are provided to meet a person's health concerns.
>
> Equity is the state whereby opportunities for health gains are available for everyone.
>
> Relevance is the degree to which most important and locally relevant problems are tackled first and most vulnerable people receive priority attention.
>
> Effectiveness ensures that greatest impact on people's health is sought, making an optimal use of available resources.

3.3.3 Social Responsibility, Social Responsiveness and Social Accountability

Social obligation includes social responsibility, social responsiveness and social accountability (Boelen et al. 2016). In social responsibility, objectives are defined by faculty, programmes are community oriented and focus of evaluation is process. In social responsiveness, objectives are defined using data, programmes are community based and focus of evaluation is outcome. In social accountability, needs and objectives are defined by collaboration with society, programmes are community engaged and focus of evaluation is impact on health needs (Boelen et al. 2016).

3.3.4 Scope of Social Accountability of Medical Schools

The scope of social accountability of medical schools is wide and includes areas of education, service and research.

3.4 Increasing Acceptance of Social Accountability in the Twenty-First Century

3.4.1 Training for Health Equity Network (THEnet)

THEnet is a network of health professional schools, located in different countries of the world, which work on the principles of social accountability (Ross et al. 2014).

3.4.2 Global Consensus for Social Accountability of Medical Schools (GCSA)

The Global Consensus for Social Accountability of Medical Schools (2010) was developed by an International Reference Group facilitated by a steering committee with the support of the World Health Organization (WHO), THEnet of medical schools, Société Internationale Francophone d'Education Médicale (SIFEM) and the World Federation for Medical Education. The Global Consensus suggests measures grouped under ten areas for improving social accountability of medical schools.

3.4.3 The Lancet Commission Report

The Lancet Commission Report suggested a new professionalism which included social accountability (Frenk et al. 2010).

3.4.4 WFME Global Standards for Quality Improvement in Basic Medical Education

WFME Global Standards for Quality Improvement in Basic Medical Education (World Federation for Medical Education 2003) included social responsibility as a quality development standard in its mission and objectives. The 2012 Revision of WFME Global Standards for Quality Improvement in Basic Medical Education (World Federation for Medical Education 2012) included social accountability in its mission as a basic standard.

3.4.5 ASPIRE Recognition of Excellence in Social Accountability of a Medical, Dental and Veterinary School

This is an initiative of the Association for Medical Education in Europe (AMEE) (2015). This uses four sets of criteria to recognize excellence in social accountability of medical schools in any country in the world. These criteria pertain to organization, education, research and health services.

3.4.6 Frameworks for Evaluation of Social Accountability of Medical Schools

Different frameworks are available for evaluation of social accountability of medical schools. Boelen et al. (2012) have described a framework based on conceptualization, production and usability with indicators of social accountability of medical schools. Ross et al. (2014) have described the Training for Health Equity Network framework for evaluation which is a practical adaptation of conceptualization-production-usability model. In ASPIRE Recognition of Excellence in Social Accountability of a medical, dental and veterinary school, evidence of plans, actions and impacts are required for evaluation (Association for Medical Education in Europe (AMEE) 2015).

3.5 Improving Social Accountability in Undergraduate Medical Education

Different undergraduate medical education programmes will vary in social accountability. Hence each medical school should decide about measures to improve social accountability of its undergraduate education programme. Global Consensus for Social Accountability of Medical Schools (2010) and ASPIRE Recognition of Excellence in Social Accountability of a Medical, Dental and Veterinary School programme (Association for Medical Education in Europe (AMEE) 2015) have described criteria for social accountability. Based on these, following measures are suggested to improve social accountability of undergraduate medical education.

3.5.1 Educational Measures

3.5.1.1 Four Values/Principles of Social Accountability

Four values/principles of quality, equity, relevance and effectiveness are essential to achieve social accountability in education.

3.5.1.2 Assessment of Health Needs in Collaboration with Stakeholders

Health needs of the geographical region assigned to the medical school should be assessed in consultation with the community and other stakeholders such as the healthcare system, medical education system (leadership, health professional teachers and students) and government regulators.

3.5.1.3 Need-Based Selection of Students

Selection of students should reflect demographic diversity and underprivileged groups of the region and those who are most likely to respond to the health needs of the community.

3.5.1.4 Focus on Social Accountability

Social accountability is part of mission statement and is the purpose of all activities in the programme.

3.5.1.5 Use of Outcome-Based Education

An outcome-based educational programme should be used. Outcomes should be derived from the health needs of the community.

3.5.1.6 Evaluation of Impact of Educational Programme on Health Needs

Graduate doctors of the educational programme should improve the quality, equity, relevance and effectiveness of healthcare received by the community.

3.5.1.7 Use of Collaboration with Stakeholders

Collaboration with stakeholders is used for effective and efficient management of educational programme.

3.5.2 General Measures

1. Coordination and cooperation between medical education and healthcare systems are to be encouraged.
2. Good governance of medical schools is essential.
3. Use of standards for internal programme evaluation and accreditation is required.
4. Continuous quality improvement philosophy is to be followed.

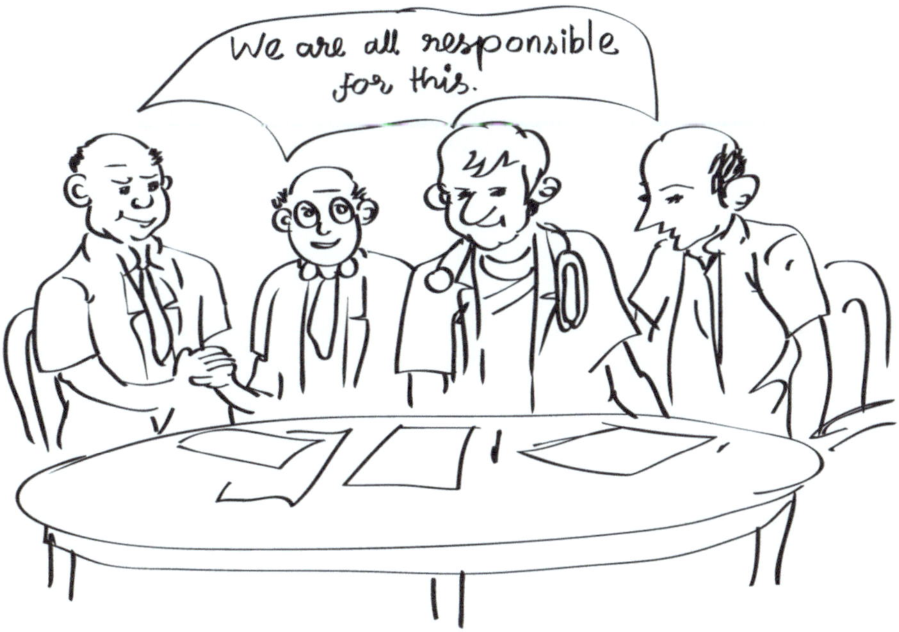

Fig. 3.2 Social accountability-collective responsibility

Conclusions

Social accountability is the purpose of medical schools. Medical schools serve the needs of the society through service, education and research. The increasingly popular concept of social accountability has the advantage of including the evaluation of impact on health needs making it possible to ensure that health needs have been fulfilled. Social accountability of undergraduate medical education can be improved by various measures including assessment of health needs in collaboration with stakeholders, need-based selection of students and use of outcome-based education.

References

Association for Medical Education in Europe (AMEE) (2015) ASPIRE Recognition of Excellence in Social Accountability of a Medical, Dental and Veterinary School. Association for Medical Education in Europe (AMEE); Jan 2015. Available from http://www.aspire-to-excellence.org/downloads/1303/ASPIRE%20Social%20Accountability%20-%20An%20Introduction_Sept%202017.pdf. Accessed 13 Jan 2018

Boelen C, Dharamsi S, Gibbs T (2012) The social accountability of medical schools and its indicators. Educ Health 25(3):180–194. https://doi.org/10.4103/1357-6283.109785 Available from http://www.educationforhealth.net/article.asp?issn=1357-6283;year=2012;volume=25;issue=3;spage=180;epage=194;aulast=Boelen. Accessed 13 Jan 2018

Boelen C, Heck JE (1995) Defining and measuring the social accountability of medical schools. World Health Organization, Geneva Available from http://apps.who.int/iris/bitstream/10665/59441/1/WHO_HRH_95.7.pdf. Accessed 13 Jan 2018

Boelen C, Pearson D, Kaufman A, Rourke J, Woollard R, Marsh DC et al (2016) Producing a socially accountable medical school: AMEE Guide No. 109. Med Teach 38(11):1078–1091. https://doi.org/10.1080/0142159X.2016.1219029 PMID: 27608933

Frenk J, Chen C, Bhutta Z, Chen J, Crisp N, Evans T et al (2010) Health professionals for a new century: transforming education to strengthen health systems in an interdependent world. Lancet 376:1923–1958. https://doi.org/10.1016/S0140-6736(10)61854-5

Global Consensus for Social Accountability of Medical Schools (2010.) Available from http://healthsocialaccountability.sites.olt.ubc.ca/files/2011/06/11-06-07-GCSA-English-pdf-style.pdf. Accessed 13 Jan 2018

Government of India (1983) National Health Policy. Ministry of Health and Family Welfare, Government of India, New Delhi Available from https://www.nhp.gov.in/sites/default/files/pdf/nhp_1983.pdf. Accessed 13 Jan 2018

Ross SJ, Preston R, Lindemann IC, Matte MC, Samson R, Tandinco FD et al (2014) The Training for Health Equity Network evaluation framework: a pilot study at five health professional schools. Educ Health 27(2):116–126. https://doi.org/10.4103/1357-6283.143727 PMID: 25420971

United Nations (1948) United Nations Universal Declaration of Human Rights. United Nations Department of Public Information. Available from http://www.un.org/en/universal-declaration-human-rights/. Accessed 13 Jan 2018

World Federation for Medical Education (2003) Basic Medical Education WFME Global Standards for Quality Improvement. WFME, Copenhagen Available from http://www.saidem.org.ar/docs/Normas/WFME.%20Global%20standards%20for%20quality%20improvement.pdf. Accessed 13 Jan 2018

World Federation for Medical Education (2012) Basic Medical Education. WFME Global Standards for Quality Improvement. The 2012 Revision. WFME, Copenhagen Available from http://www.um.es/documents/1935287/1936044/Revision_of_Standards_ for_Basic_Medical_Education_FINAL_260912.pdf/5866f7af-f7fc-4f9a-a7e6-eb054b7795c3. Accessed 8 Jan 2018

World Federation for Medical Education (1988) The Edinburgh Declaration. Lancet 8068:464

World Health Organization (2006) Constitution of the World Health Organization. World Health Organization, basic documents, 45th edn. Supplement, Oct 2006. Available from http://www.who.int/governance/eb/who_constitution_en.pdf. Accessed 13 Jan 2018

World Health Organization (1981) Global Strategy for Health for All by the Year 2000. World Health Organization, Geneva Available from http://apps.who.int/iris/bitstream/10665/38893/1/9241800038.pdf. Accessed 13 Jan 2018

World Health Organization (1988) Reorientation of Medical Education: goals, strategies and targets (2). World Health Organization Regional Office for South-East Asia, New Delhi

Basics of Curriculum and Curriculum Change

4

Objectives

1. Define a curriculum and discuss the need for planning and for curriculum.
2. List components of a curriculum document along with their main features.
3. Describe curriculum approaches and non-formal curricula.
4. Discuss curriculum determinants and curriculum planning and curriculum management approaches.
5. Discuss implementation challenges, obstacles and facilitators of curriculum change.
6. Describe cyclical problem-solving research-based approach to curriculum change and continuous improvement of undergraduate medical curriculum.

4.1 Introduction

As part of social accountability, medical schools should adapt their undergraduate educational programme to the health needs of the society. The educational programme should keep responding to the health needs of the society because the health needs keep changing. In other words, the educational programme should be dynamic and not be static. The World Federation for Medical Education (WFME) Global Standards for Quality Improvement in Basic Medical Education (2012) have emphasized the need for continuous renewal in basic medical education. Dolmans et al. (2011) have suggested that there should be continuous improvement of medical education. The principle of continuous improvement is well accepted in service

Kadambari D et al., *Improving Discipline-Based Undergraduate Medical Curriculum*, https://doi.org/10.1007/978-981-13-1310-3_4

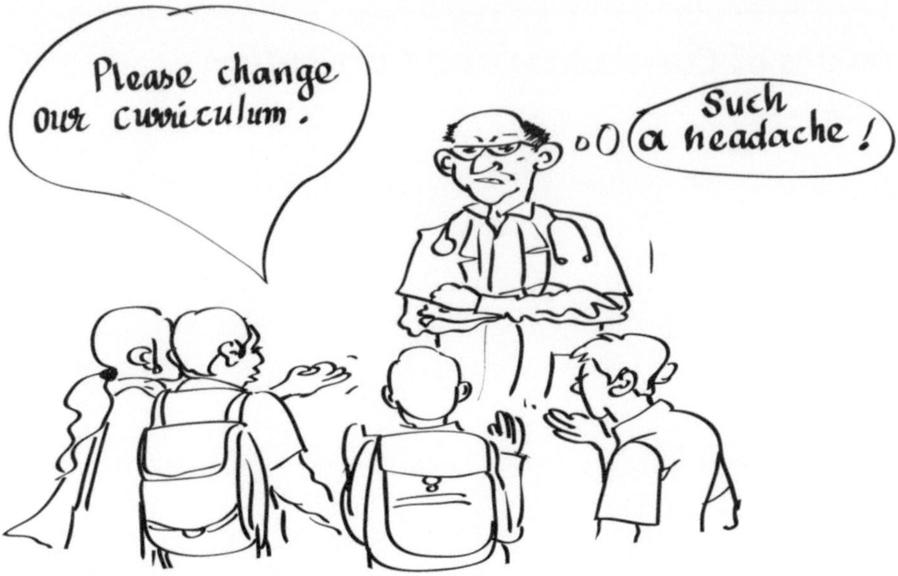

Fig. 4.1 Reluctance for curriculum change

(patient care) and research. The same principle needs to be applied consistently in education. Curriculum is the means to improve educational programmes. In this chapter, initial portions deal with various features of undergraduate medical curriculum, and later portions deal with curriculum change with the ultimate purpose of continuous improvement.

4.2 Why Should We Plan?

> Failing to plan is planning to fail.
> Benjamin Franklin

Before doing anything, usually we decide what is to be done (goal/objective/outcome) and how it should be done. In other words, we plan before doing anything. The better we plan, the more the chances of succeeding. As in any field of endeavour, planning is essential in health profession also. In service side of health profession, we make management plans for patients. In health professional research, plans are called research proposals. In health professional education, planning is equally important, and plans for educational programmes are called curricula. All educational programmes, courses and sessions should be planned and should have plans or curricula. Unplanned educational activities have lower chances of success.

4.3 What Is a Curriculum?

A curriculum is a formal plan for conducting an educational programme in an educational institution. An undergraduate medical curriculum is a formal plan for undergraduate medical educational programme in an institution. An undergraduate programme involves more than one discipline. Hence planning and implementing undergraduate curriculum are more complex and challenging than managing a postgraduate curriculum which involves only one discipline.

4.4 Components of a Curriculum Document

As a curriculum is useful only to the extent it is implemented, the curriculum document should include an implementation plan. In addition, an evaluation plan is also needed for finding out whether the implementation is adequate. The components of a curriculum document are planned by a curriculum committee with the participation of leadership and faculty members. These components should include the following.

4.4.1 Curriculum

4.4.1.1 Purposes of the Programme

Purposes should include basic reasons for having the undergraduate medical educational programme. These can include social accountability and important qualities of doctors to be produced.

4.4.1.2 Outcomes

Outcomes are results of learning that doctors need to possess. Outcomes should be wide, long and deep (Hamilton 1999).

4.4.1.3 Content (Syllabus)

Content includes knowledge, attitudes and skills to be learnt to achieve outcomes.

4.4.1.4 Learning

Learning includes all processes which will help in learning.

4.4.1.5 Assessment

Assessment includes all processes which will help in knowing that learning has occurred. It will include formative and summative assessments.

4.4.1.6 Organization and Scheduling

Plans are made for organizing and scheduling of learning and assessment processes.

4.4.1.7 Resources Required

Resources required include faculty, space, equipment, money and time.

4.4.2 Curriculum Implementation Plan

Curriculum committee should make detailed plans for faculty, space, equipment, money and time requirements, leadership support, faculty development programmes, learning resource development, monitoring of implementation and formative evaluation of the programme. Monitoring of implementation and formative evaluation are needed for support and for course correction if necessary.

4.4.3 Programme Evaluation Plan

Evaluation of programme includes formative evaluation and summative evaluation. Curriculum committee should make detailed plan for formative and summative programme evaluation.

4.5 Why Is a Curriculum Needed?

A curriculum is a written plan available to teachers, students and other stakeholders. A curriculum guides teachers for carrying out various roles of a teacher. Students are guided in their learning efforts by a curriculum which is well written and transparent. One-third of the learning of students is from formal or declared curriculum, one-third of learning is from taught curriculum and one-third of learning is from hidden curriculum (Harden 2013). Thus an effective curriculum document should promote self-learning and self-reliance in students.

4.6 Curriculum Approaches in Undergraduate Medical Education

Papa and Harasym (1999) described five curriculum approaches as they have evolved in North America from the viewpoint of cognitive science. These approaches in order of their evolution in North America are briefly described below.

4.6.1 Apprenticeship-Based Approach

In this approach, content is organized around subjects and controlled by faculty, and teaching method is lecture (Papa and Harasym 1999).

4.6.2 Discipline-Based Approach

In discipline-based approach, content is organized around disciplines and controlled by departments, and teaching method is lecture (Papa and Harasym 1999). In discipline-based approach, courses are identified by the names of disciplines such as anatomy, physiology, etc. in the first year and pathology, pharmacology, etc. in the second year (Hecker and Violato 2008).

4.6.3 System-Based Approach

In this approach, content is organized around organ systems and controlled by the topic committee, and the main teaching method is lecture (Papa and Harasym 1999). System-based approach may be either used only in the second year or both in first and second years (Hecker and Violato 2008). In system-based approach, courses are identified by names of organ systems such as respiratory, cardiovascular, etc.

4.6.4 Problem-Based Approach

In problem-based approach, content is organized around clinical cases and controlled by the curriculum committee, and the main teaching method is small groups (Papa and Harasym 1999).

4.6.5 Clinical Presentation-Based Approach

In this approach, content is organized around clinical presentations and controlled by the curriculum committee, and lecture and small groups are equally used as teaching methods (Papa and Harasym 1999).

In the study of Hecker and Violato (2008), curriculum approaches in the medical schools of the United States from 1992 to 1999 were described.

- Discipline-based approach was used by 65.5% of schools in 1992 and by 40.5% in 1999.
- Problem-based approach was employed by 10.3% of schools in 1992 and by 25% in 1999.
- Organ system-based approach only in the second year was used by 12.1% of schools in 1992 and by 17.2% in 1999.
- Organ system-based approach both in first and second years was employed by 5.2% of schools in 1992 and by 10.3% in 1999.
- Other approaches were used by 6.9% of schools in 1992 and by 6.9% in 1999.

Thus the use of discipline-based approach decreased, and the use of other three named approaches increased from 1992 to 1999 in the United States.

In India, discipline-based approach has remained the commonest in undergraduate medical education (Supe and Burdick 2006).

4.7 Non-Formal Curricula

Hafferty and Gaufberg (2013) classified curricula into four types: formal, informal, hidden and null. Formal curriculum is what is given in the curriculum document or conveyed by teachers. Informal curriculum includes learning from interactions with teachers, peers and others. Hidden curriculum is learning from institutional norms and practices. Null curriculum involves learning from what is not covered or emphasized in the formal curriculum. For example, if social accountability is not covered, it may be considered unimportant. Informal and hidden curricula may or may not be aligned to the formal curriculum. Methods have been described to assess non-formal curricula (Hafferty and Gaufberg (2013). Non-formal curricula are parts of the educational environment. Balmer et al. (2013) used the classification of explicit curriculum, implicit curriculum and extracurriculum in their study. Explicit curriculum was formal curriculum, implicit curriculum included informal and hidden curricula and extracurriculum included learning from activities such as volunteering. In their study, students perceived that learning of knowledge and skills occurred mainly in explicit curriculum. Extracurriculum was useful for learning about self-awareness and new knowledge. Implicit curriculum was important for learning about commitment to patients, communication, teamwork, teaching, lifelong learning and deep understanding of patients. In implicit curriculum, observation played an important role in learning. Implicit curriculum may or may not support the intended formal curriculum.

4.8 Curriculum Determinants

Curriculum determinants are the factors that should determine the curriculum. Curriculum determinants can be described under the following groups.

4.8.1 Health Needs of the Society

As per the concept of social accountability, health needs of the society are the primary curriculum determinants. These direct the choice of other curriculum determinants. Health needs of the society can be understood from the following resources.

4.8.1.1 National Health Policy

Situation Analyses: Backdrop to the National Health Policy 2017 (Government of India 2017a, b) described situation in various areas including achievements in Millennium Development Goals, burden of disease, human resource development and investment in healthcare. National Health Policy 2017 (Government of India

2017a, b) included in its goal the attainment of universal health coverage of good quality without financial hardship. It prescribed policy in various areas including medical education in which the following is included:

> The policy recognizes the need to revise the undergraduate and postgraduate medical curriculum keeping in view the changing needs, technology and the newer emerging disease trends.

4.8.1.2 Global Recommendations

The World Health Report 2008: Primary Health Care—Now More than Ever (World Health Organization 2008) emphasized the need for primary healthcare and gave suggestions for reforms. Sustainable Development Goals (United Nations 2015) described health needs under Goal 3. 'Ensure healthy lives and promote well-being for all at all ages'. Goal 3.8 included 'Achieve universal health coverage, including financial risk protection….'

4.8.2 Professional Service Requirements

For fulfilling healthcare needs of the society, medical graduates should demonstrate certain learning outcomes. Several outcome frameworks are available and are listed under the following categories.

4.8.2.1 National Outcome Frameworks

(a) The Roles of the Indian Medical Graduate.

The roles of the Indian Medical Graduate include clinician, leader and member of the healthcare team and system, communicator, lifelong learner and professional (Medical Council of India's Regulations on Graduate Medical Education—Proposed 2012). These roles include competencies, and the total number of competencies is 35.

(b) General Medical Council (UK) Outcomes.

The General Medical Council, UK (2015), recommends outcomes under three roles of the doctor: as a scholar and a scientist, as a practitioner and as a professional. There are a total of 16 outcomes under these three roles. These 16 outcomes include 106 smaller outcomes.

(c) Accreditation Council for Graduate Medical Education or ACGME (USA) Competencies.

ACGME competencies are grouped under the categories of patient care and procedural skills, medical knowledge, practice-based learning and improvement, interpersonal and communication skills, professionalism and systems-based practice (Accreditation Council for Graduate Medical Education 2017).

(d) The CanMEDS Physician Competency Framework (Canada).

The CanMEDS Physician Competency Framework includes the roles of medical expert, communicator, collaborator, leader, health advocate, scholar and professional (Frank et al. 2015).

4.8.2.2 Global Outcome Frameworks

(a) Global Minimum Essential Requirements.

The Core Committee of Institute for International Medical Education (2002) grouped 60 essential requirements under seven outcome-competence categories of (1) professional values, attitudes, behaviour and ethics, (2) scientific foundations of medicine, (3) communication skills, (4) clinical skills, (5) population health and health systems, (6) management of information and (7) critical thinking and research.

(b) The Roles of the Doctor in WFME Global Standards.

WFME Global Standards for Quality Improvement in Basic Medical Education mentioned the roles of the doctor as scholar and scientist, practitioner, communicator, teacher, manager and professional (World Federation for Medical Education 2012). In addition, the role of lifelong learner was also indicated. Other important outcomes pertained to behavioural sciences, patient safety and evidence-based medicine.

4.8.2.3 Other Frameworks

(a) The Scottish Doctor Framework of Learning Outcomes.

It was based on three essential elements of 'what the doctor is able to do,' 'how the doctor approaches his/her practice' and 'the doctor as professional' as part of a three-circle model (Scottish Deans' Medical Education Group 2008). The three essential elements included 12 domains of learning outcomes.

(b) The Nine Abilities of the Warren Alpert Medical School of Brown University (USA).

The Warren Alpert Medical School of Brown University (2017) has used nine abilities of effective communication, basic clinical skills, using basic science in the practice of medicine, diagnosis, prevention and treatment, lifelong learning, professionalism, community health advocacy and promotion, medical ethics and moral reasoning and clinical decision-making.

4.8.3 Professional Educational Requirements

These are contained in following resources.

4.8.3.1 Medical Council of India's Recommendations

Professional educational requirements are available in Medical Council of India's Regulations on Graduate Medical Education (1997) and its amendments and Medical Council of India's Regulations on Graduate Medical Education—Proposed (2012).

4.8.3.2 Global Resources

Professional educational requirements are covered in detail in WFME Global Standards for Quality Improvement in Basic Medical Education (World Federation for Medical Education 2012).

SPICES model (Harden et al. 1984) has been popular for deciding educational strategies in curriculum planning. Each letter of SPICES stands for the preferable end of a continuum. These continua are teacher-centred to student-centred, information-oriented to problem-oriented, isolated to integrated, hospital-based to community-based, standard programme to electives and opportunistic to systematic. PRISMS is another model of strategies to guide curriculum planning (Bligh et al. 2001). P stands for product-focused, R for relevant, I for interprofessional, S for shorter courses and smaller numbers, M for multisite and S for symbiotic. Thus the curriculum should be product-focused using learning outcomes, relevant to societal needs and symbiotic involving health and education systems. Other features are the use of shorter courses and smaller groups for learning, interprofessional learning and primary and secondary care settings for learning.

4.8.4 Resources Available

Choice of professional service and educational requirements have to be carefully balanced with resources available. Resources include faculty, space, equipment, money and time.

4.9 Forward and Backward Approaches to Curriculum Planning

Curriculum can be planned using forward and backward approaches (Smith 2009). Functional stages of systems approach (Input → Process → Output) can be used for understanding these approaches.

4.9.1 Forward Planning of Curriculum

In forward planning of curriculum, input or content drives the curriculum following the Input → Process → Output sequence. This approach is usually associated with traditional discipline-based curriculum.

4.9.2 Backward Planning of Curriculum

In backward planning of curriculum, outcomes drive the curriculum reversing the Input → Process → Output sequence. The outcomes determine the content, learning and assessment. This approach is associated with outcome-based education (Harden et al. 1999).

4.10 Departmental and Central Approaches to Managing Undergraduate Curriculum

Undergraduate medical curriculum can be managed and controlled using departmental and central approaches which are described below.

4.10.1 Departmental Approach

Departmental approach to managing is associated with traditional discipline-based curriculum. In this approach, departments of disciplines involved in undergraduate medical education are delegated with all responsibilities of undergraduate education except admissions and summative assessments which are controlled by central academic management. Advantages of departmental approach include use of existing departmental organizational structure and teaching by experts in various disciplines. Limitations of departmental approach include underemphasis on the outcomes of undergraduate curriculum and lack of accountability for these outcomes (Reynolds III et al. 1995).

4.10.2 Central Approach

WFME Global Standards for Quality Improvement in Basic Medical Education (World Federation for Medical Education 2012) recommends that there must be a curriculum committee, under the academic leadership, responsible for planning and implementation of undergraduate medical curriculum. The curriculum committee must ensure that required learning outcomes are achieved by graduating students. The advantages of central curriculum committee are that curriculum learning outcomes are emphasized and interdisciplinary areas are adequately covered. The limitation of curriculum committee is that it involves use of more resources. An amendment of Medical Council of India's Regulations on Graduate Medical Education (1997) requires that there should be a curriculum committee in every medical college in India for regular updating of curriculum.

4.11 Curriculum Change: The Challenge of Implementation

The implementation of undergraduate medical curriculum has always been challenging. Two types of implementation gaps can occur.

1. Gap between committee recommendations and formal curriculum
2. Gap between formal curriculum and taught curriculum

These two gaps are described below.

4.11.1 Gap Between Committee Recommendations and Formal Curriculum

The Lancet Commission Report (Frenk et al. 2010) has referred to 'fragmented, outdated and static curricula' which are unable to respond to health needs of the society. This curriculum stasis is responsible for the implementation gap between committee recommendations and formal curriculum. Medical Council of India's Minimum Recommendations on Graduate Medical Education (1981) referred to the problem of implementation in the following words:

> Deficiencies which exist at present, if any, are attributable more to a failure of implementation of Council recommendations and the absence of a system of continuous monitoring of the training scheme.

In the United States, Educating Medical Students: Assessing Change in Medical Education—The Road to Implementation or The ACME-TRI Report (Swanson and Anderson 1993) included the following:

> ...most medical schools have done little to correct the major shortcomings in the ways they educate their students, even though these deficiencies have been documented repeatedly.

The General Medical Council, UK, in *Tomorrow's Doctors* (1993) had referred to 'the persistent gap between the good intentions of successive Councils and the implementation of their recommendations'.

An idea about the extent of implementation gap can be had from the following citations. Regan-Smith (1998) noted that learning of problem-solving and critical thinking recommended in the *Flexner Report* had not been widely implemented. Harden (1998) observed that problem-based learning and Objective Structured Clinical Examination had taken more than 25 years to be adopted. Lack of use of MCQs in assessment is another indicator of implementation gap.

However, the implementation of reforms has started improving from the 1990s in response to an emphasis on accountability and accreditation as a result of the publication of the Edinburgh Declaration (World Federation for Medical Education 1988), *Tomorrow's Doctors* (General Medical Council 1993), Education Medical Students: Assessing Change in Medical Education, The Road to Implementation or The ACME, TRI Report (Swanson and Anderson 1993) and other recommendations and the efforts of governments.

Reforms in educational programmes in the United States and Canada have been documented in snapshot reports from medical schools (Anderson 2000; Anderson and Kanter 2010). In a summary of Snapshot Reports (2010) from 128 medical schools in the United States and Canada, significant changes have been mentioned under categories of curriculum management and governance structure, office of medical education, financial management of educational programmes, valuing teaching, curriculum renewal process, learning outcomes/competencies, new topics in the curriculum, advances in pedagogy, advances in assessment, clinical experiences and regional campus (Anderson and Kanter 2010).

In the United Kingdom, reforms in undergraduate medical education since the publication of *Tomorrow's Doctors* (General Medical Council 1993) included the use of core curriculum and special study modules, integrated courses and student-centred approach (Harden et al. 2002).

In a survey including 849 responses from 73 countries, 7 major curriculum trends were identified from a global perspective (Kennedy et al. 2012). This survey was undertaken by MEDINE 2 Work Package 5 Taskforce and Association of Medical Education in Europe (AMEE). These major trends were the use of MCQs, curriculum committee, learning in small groups, clinical skills unit, inclusion of communication skills in outcomes, emphasis on attitudes and professionalism along with knowledge and skills and drug prescribing as an outcome. Minor trends included a curriculum based on well-defined learning outcomes; use of learning outcomes in deciding content, teaching methods and assessment; opportunities for students to go abroad for study; an increase in number of students admitted; use of ambulatory care settings for training and the use of OSCE in assessment.

An effective accreditation process is required as an initiator for widespread improvement of reform process in undergraduate medical educational programme in India (Supe and Burdick 2006; Sood 2008; Amin et al. 2010).

4.11.2 Gap Between Formal Curriculum and Taught Curriculum

The formal or declared curriculum is only partly taught (Harden 2013), creating an implementation gap.

4.12 Curriculum Change: Obstacles

In a worldwide survey involving 1006 respondents from 92 countries, obstacles to change in curriculum were identified under four groups (Kennedy et al. 2012). Group 'Status quo' included factors of culture of conservatism and satisfaction with the current approach. Group 'Proposed change' included factors of teachers not convinced that change will lead to an improvement and not trained to implement the change. Group 'Cost of change' included factors of increased workload of planning and implementing the change and lack of resources for change. Group 'Process of change' included factors of teachers' work not incentivized or rewarded and teachers' conflicting interests of research and clinical care.

The factors under 'Process of change' listed above were ranked highest as major obstacles in closed survey and were also included among the main obstacles in open response survey.

Fear of loss of control by teachers in an important obstacle in introducing change in lecture-based and teacher-centred curriculum (Mennin and Kaufman 1989). In teacher-centred approach, teachers are used to having full control over content and teaching methods. Hence, a curriculum change, which usually involves a shift to student-centred approach and more control to students, results in concerns for teachers. Teachers who have studied in the existing system start believing in the system due to socialization effect (Mennin and Kaufman 1989). This may explain liking and support for status quo.

4.13 Curriculum Change: Facilitators

In a literature review, Bland et al. (2000) identified leadership, human resource development (including training support and reward structure), politics, cooperative climate, evaluation and participation by organization members as factors most important for success in curriculum change. Leadership was found to be the most essential for curriculum change because it can influence all other necessary factors. Leadership can also help in overcoming obstacles described earlier.

As teachers and students are the stakeholders who will implement the planned change, it is essential that they develop ownership for change by their participation in problem identification and planning stages. Ownership is developed if the concepts and principles of problem and planned change are shared with teachers and students and their inputs are sought and accepted (Mennin and Kaufman 1989).

Treating change intervention as an experimental research study and thorough longitudinal programme evaluation increases its credibility and acceptability among teachers (Mennin and Kaufman 1989).

4.14 Cyclical Problem-Solving Research-Based Approach to Curriculum Change

Three main principles of cyclical problem-solving research-based approach to curriculum change are given below.

4.14.1 Cyclical Approach

It is making small changes on a regular basis. Curriculum change consists of repeated cycles of change. This is based on a management concept for improvement called Deming cycle or PDCA cycle or Plan-Do-Check-Act cycle (Kanji and Asher 1996). For continuous improvement this cycle should be used repeatedly. Plan stage includes identifying a problem, finding out the causes of the problem and making a plan to solve the problem. This concept is often used in medical profession. For example, when we treat a patient, there is identifying of patient problems, making a diagnosis and making a treatment plan ('plan' stage), implementing the plan ('do' stage), evaluating the treatment ('check' stage) and acting on evaluation results, i.e. continuing the plan or modifying the plan ('act' stage).

4.14.2 Problem-Solving Approach

The purpose of change is problem-solving. Problem is identified before and separately from the planning of solutions. This happens when diagnosis is separated from treatment in patient care. Separate identification of problem before planning of solutions has been recommended in curriculum change (Gale and Grant 1997). Identification of problem and getting agreement on the problem by teachers helps in building ownership (Gale and Grant 1997).

4.14.3 Research-Based Approach

As mentioned earlier, if change intervention is carried out as an experimental research study with longitudinal programme evaluation, the process becomes scientific and more acceptable by teachers (Mennin and Kaufman 1989).

4.15 One Cycle of Problem-Solving Research-Based Approach to Curriculum Change

It can have the following steps.

4.15.1 Ensuring Availability of Facilitators of Curriculum Change

Facilitators of curriculum change described earlier including leadership support and guidance and faculty development facilities should be available to support change. A curriculum committee should also be available to manage the change.

4.15.2 Analysing Situation and Defining Problems

Appropriate research approach should be used to identify problems in educational processes (outcomes, content, learning and assessment) keeping in view societal health needs, service requirements and educational requirements. The evidence about the problems is discussed with teachers and students, and agreement is reached about educational problems.

4.15.3 Planning Solutions

Solutions for identified problems are sought from educational literature and are discussed with teachers and students. Views and inputs of teachers and students are sought about the solutions with evidence from the literature. Their inputs are considered and accepted if necessary to encourage development of ownership.

Planning should include making plan for solutions, making implementation plan and making plan for evaluating change being implemented.

4.15.4 Implementing the Plan

The plan is implemented and help and support are provided during the implementation. Formative evaluation is done as part of monitoring of implementation to provide reinforcement and any corrective action if necessary.

4.15.5 Evaluating Change

Formative and summative evaluation of change will help in indicating whether the change has led to the solution of the problems.

4.15.6 Acting on Evaluation Results

If evaluation results show that the change has led to the desired improvement, the change is reinforced and continued. If desired improvement has not occurred, corrective steps will be necessary as part of next cycle of change.

4.16 Continuous Improvement of Undergraduate Medical Curriculum

Continuous improvement of undergraduate medical curriculum is required for continuous improvement of undergraduate medical educational programme in response to continuously changing health needs, service requirements and educational requirements.

Repeated cycles of problem-solving research-based approach should be used for continuous improvement of undergraduate medical curriculum.

India's MBBS programme (Medical Council of India's Regulations on Graduate Medical Education 1997) has the following five courses.

	Course	Duration
1.	Phase I	1 year
2.	Phase II	1.5 years
3.	Phase III part 1	1 year
4.	Phase III part 2	1 year
5.	Internship	1 year

Each course consists of short sessions of theory, practical, clinical and field visit held everyday. Thus opportunities for improvement at session level are available everyday. Course-level opportunities for improvement are available five times for every batch. Programme-level improvement can be carried out once for every batch. If these opportunities are used for improvement of curriculum, continuous improvement of undergraduate medical curriculum can be done.

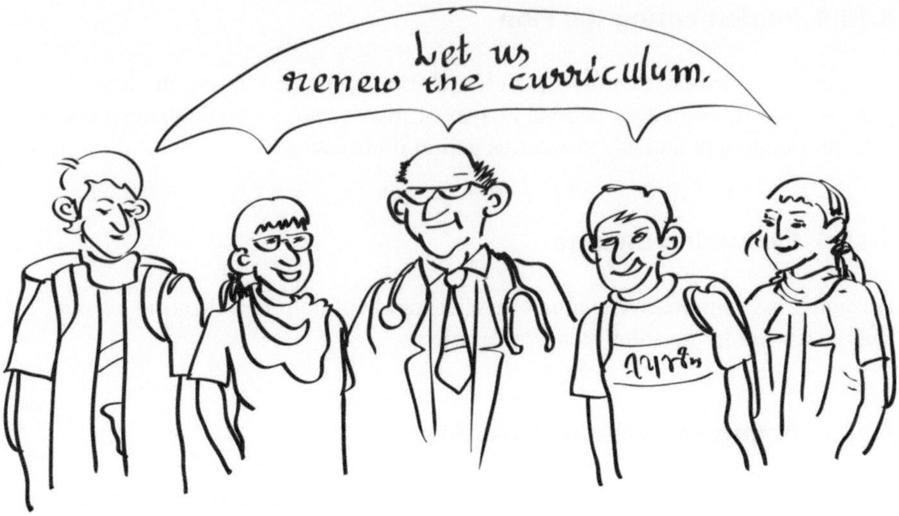

Fig. 4.2 Acceptance of curriculum change

Conclusions

Curriculum is an instrument to translate societal health needs, professional service requirements and educational requirements into students' learning. A curriculum should be dynamic to serve the changing health needs of the society and evolving service and educational requirements. Curriculum change need not be a one-time affair. Small changes on a regular basis can lead to continuous improvement of undergraduate medical curriculum. A cyclical problem-solving research-based approach is preferable for curriculum change. Curriculum change is challenging but possible with leadership support and faculty development programmes.

References

Accreditation Council for Graduate Medical Education (2017) ACGME. Common programme requirements. Available from https://www.acgme.org/Portals/0/PFAssets/ProgramRequirements/CPRs_2017-07-01.pdf. Accessed 13 Jan 2018

Amin Z, Burdick WP, Supe A, Singh T (2010) Relevance of the Flexner Report to contemporary medical education in South Asia. Acad Med 85(2):333–339. https://doi.org/10.1097/ACM.0b013e3181c874cb Available from http://journals.lww.com/academicmedicine/Abstract/2010/02000/Relevance_of_the_Flexner_Report_to_Contemporary.36.aspx. Accessed 13 Jan 2018

Anderson MB (2000) A guide to the 130 reports in this Snapshot Supplement to Academic Medicine. Acad Med 75(9, September Suppl):Sx–Sxiv Available from http://journals.lww.com/academicmedicine/Citation/2000/09001/A_Guide_to_the_130_Reports_in_This_Snapshot.2.aspx. Accessed 13 Jan 2018

Anderson MB, Kanter SL (2010) Medical education in the United States and Canada, 2010. Acad Med 85(9, September Suppl):S2–S18. PMID: 20736548. https://doi.org/10.1097/ACM.0b013e3181f16f52

Balmer DF, Hall E, Fink M, Richards BF (2013) How do medical students navigate the interplay of explicit curricula, implicit curricula, and extracurricula to learn curricular objectives? Acad Med 88(8):1135–1141. https://doi.org/10.1097/ACM.0b013e31829a6c39 Available from http://journals.lww.com/academicmedicine/Abstract/2013/08000/How_Do_Medical_Students_Navigate_the_Interplay_of.32.aspx. Accessed 13 Jan 2018

Bland CJ, Starnaman S, Wersal L, Moorhead-Rosenberg L, Zonia S, Henry R (2000) Curricular change in medical schools: how to succeed. Acad Med 75(6):575–594 Available from http://citeseerx.ist.psu.edu/viewdoc/download?doi=10.1.1.494.5008&rep=rep1&type=pdf. Accessed 13 Jan 2018

Bligh J, Prideaux D, Parsell G (2001) PRISMS: new educational strategies for medical education. Med Educ 35:520–521. https://doi.org/10.1046/j.1365-2923.2001.00984.x Available from http://onlinelibrary.wiley.com/doi/10.1046/j.1365-2923.2001.00984.x/abstract. Accessed 13 Jan 2018

Core Committee, Institute for International Medical Education (2002) Global minimum essential requirements in medical education. Med Teach 24(2):130–135. PMID: 12098431. https://doi.org/10.1080/01421590220120731

Dolmans D, Stalmeijer R, van Berkel H, Wolfhagen I (2011) Quality assurance of teaching and learning: enhancing the quality culture. In: Dornan T, Mann K, Scherpbier A, Spencer J (eds) Medical education: theory and practice. Churchill Livingstone Elsevier, Edinburgh, pp 257–264

Frank JR, Snell L, Sherbino J (eds) (2015) CanMEDS 2015 physician competency framework. Royal College of Physicians and Surgeons of Canada, Ottawa Available from www.royalcollege.ca/rcsite/documents/canmeds/canmeds-full-framework-e.pdf. Accessed 8 Jan 2018

Frenk J, Chen C, Bhutta Z, Chen J, Crisp N, Evans T et al (2010) Health professionals for a new century: transforming education to strengthen health systems in an interdependent world. Lancet 376:1923–1958. https://doi.org/10.1016/S0140-6736(10)61854-5

Gale R, Grant J (1997) AMEE Medical Education Guide No. 10: managing change in a medical context: guidelines for action. Med Teach 19(4):239–249. https://doi.org/10.3109/01421599709034200

General Medical Council (1993) Tomorrow's Doctors. Recommendations on undergraduate medical education, Dec 1993

General Medical Council (2015) Outcomes for graduates (Tomorrow's Doctors), July 2015. Available from https://www.gmc-uk.org/Outcomes_for_graduates_Jul_15_1216.pdf_61408029.pdf. Accessed 8 Jan 2018

Government of India (2017a) National Health Policy – 2017. Ministry of Health and Family Welfare, Government of India. Available from http://cdsco.nic.in/writereaddata/National-Health-Policy.pdf. Accessed 13 Jan 2018

Government of India (2017b) Situation analyses: backdrop to the National Health Policy – 2017. Ministry of Health and Family Welfare, Government of India. Available from https://mohfw.gov.in/sites/default/files/71275472221489753307.pdf. Accessed 13 Jan 2018

Hafferty FW, Gaufberg E (2013) The hidden curriculum. In: Dent JA, Harden RM (eds) A practical guide for medical teachers, 4th edn. Churchill Livingstone Elsevier, London, pp 52–58

Hamilton JD (1999) Outcomes in medical education must be wide, long and deep. Med Teach 21(2):125–126. https://doi.org/10.1080/01421599979725

Harden RM (1998) Change – building windmills not walls. Med Teach 20(3):189–191. https://doi.org/10.1080/01421599880896

Harden RM, Crosby JR, Davis MH (1999) AMEE Guide No. 14: Outcome-based education: Part 1-An introduction to outcome-based education. Med Teach 21(1): 7-14. Available from http://www.archive.jfn.ac.lk/OBESCL/MOHE/OBE-Articles/Academic-documents-articles/8.OBE-Harden-Crosby-Davis.pdf. Accessed 13 Jan 2018.

Harden RM (2013) Curriculum planning and development. In: Dent JA, Harden RM (eds) A practical guide for medical teachers, 4th edn. Churchill Livingstone Elsevier, London, pp 8–15

Harden RM, Sowden S, Dunn WR (1984) Educational strategies in curriculum development: the SPICES model. Med Educ 18:284–297 Available from https://amee.org/getattachment/AMEE-Initiatives/ESME-Courses/AMEE-ESME-Face-to-Face-Courses/ESME/ESME-Online-Resources-China-Dec-2015-(1)/Session-2-Some-educational-strategies-SPICES-Model.pdf. Accessed 13 Jan 2018

Harden RM, Davis MH, Friedman Ben-David M (2002) UK recommendations on undergraduate medical education and the Flying Wallendas. Med Teach 24(1):5–8. PMID: 12098449. https://doi.org/10.1080/00034980120103423

Hecker K, Violato C (2008) How much do differences in medical schools influence student performance? A longitudinal study employing hierarchical linear modeling. Teach Learn Med 20(2):104–113. https://doi.org/10.1080/10401330801991915

Kanji GK, Asher M (1996) Management methods. In: Kanji GK, Asher M (eds) 100 methods for total quality management. Response Books, New Delhi, pp 20–78

Kennedy C, Lilley P, Kiss L, Littvay L, Harden R (2012) MEDINE2 Work Package 5. Curriculum trends in medical education in Europe in the 21st century. Dundee, AMEE Available from http://docplayer.net/3889709-Medine2-work-package-5-curriculum-trends-in-medical-education-in-europe-in-the-21-st-century.html. Accessed 13 Jan 2018

Medical Council of India (1981) Minimum recommendations of the Medical Council of India on graduate medical education

Medical Council of India (1997) Regulations on graduate medical education. Available from https://www.mciindia.org/documents/rulesAndRegulations/GME_REGULA TIONS.pdf. Accessed 8 Jan 2018

Medical Council of India (2012) Regulations on graduate medical education – proposed. Available from http://iafmonline.in/data/circular-notifications/Revised-GME-2012.pdf. Accessed 8 Jan 2018

Mennin SP, Kaufman A (1989) The change process and medical education. Med Teach 11(1):9–16. https://doi.org/10.3109/01421598909146271

Papa FJ, Harasym PH (1999) Medical curriculum reform in North America, 1765 to the present: a cognitive science perspective. Acad Med 74(2):154–164 PMID: 10065057. Available from https://www.ncbi.nlm.nih.gov/pubmed/10065057. Accessed 13 Jan 2018

Regan-Smith MG (1998) "Reform without change": update, 1998. Acad Med 73(5):505–507 Available from http://journals.lww.com/academicmedicine/abstract/1998/05000/_reform_without_change___update,_1998.14.aspx. Accessed 13 Jan 2018

Reynolds IIICF, Adler S, Kanter SL, Horn JP, Harvey J, Bernier GM Jr (1995) The undergraduate medical curriculum; centralized versus departmentalized. Acad Med 70(8):671–675 Available from http://journals.lww.com/academicmedicine/abstract/1995/08000/the_undergraduate_medical_curriculum__centralized.7.aspx. Accessed 13 Jan 2018

Scottish Deans' Medical Education Group (2008) The Scottish Doctor. Learning outcomes for the medical undergraduate in Scotland: a foundation for competent and reflective practitioners, 3rd edn. Association for Medical Education in Europe (AMEE), Dundee Available from http://www.scottishdoctor.org/resources/scotdoc3.pdf. Accessed 8 Jan 2018

Smith SR (2009) Outcome-based curriculum. In: Dent JA, Harden RM (eds) A practical guide for medical teachers, 3rd edn. Churchill Livingstone Elsevier, Edinburgh, pp 161–167

Sood R (2008) Medical education in India. Med Teach 30:585–591. PMID: 18677660. https://doi.org/10.1080/01421590802139823

Supe A, Burdick WP (2006) Challenges and issues in medical education in India. Acad Med 81(12):1076–1080. PMID: 17122473. https://doi.org/10.1097/01.ACM.0000246699.94234.ab

Swanson AG, Anderson MB (1993) The ACME-TRI Report. Educating medical students: assessing change in medical education – the road to implementation. Acad Med 68(6, Suppl):S1–S46 Available from http://journals.lww.com/academicmedicine/Abstract/1993/06000/Educating_medical_students_Assessing_change_in.14.aspx. Accessed 13 Jan 2018

The Warren Alpert Medical School of Brown University (2017) The nine abilities. Brown University, Providence, RI Available from https://bulletin.brown.edu/medical-school/. Accessed 13 Jan 2018

United Nations (2015) Transforming our world: the 2030 agenda for sustainable development. Available from https://sustainabledevelopment.un.org/post2015/transformingourworld. Accessed 13 Jan 2018

World Federation for Medical Education (1988) The Edinburgh declaration. Lancet 8068:464

World Federation for Medical Education (2012) Basic medical education. WFME Global Standards for quality improvement. The 2012 revision. WFME, Copenhagen Available from http://www.um.es/documents/1935287/1936044/Revision_of_Standards_ for_Basic_Medical_Education_FINAL_260912.pdf/5866f7af-f7fc-4f9a-a7e6-eb054b7795c3. Accessed 8 Jan 2018

World Health Organization (2008) The world health report 2008: primary health care now more than ever. World Health Organization, Geneva Available from http://www.who.int/whr/2008/en/. Accessed 13 Jan 2018

Use of Technology

5

Objectives

1. List various global and national recommendations for the use of technology.
2. Discuss advantages, disadvantages and effectiveness of the use of technology.
3. Describe blended learning.
4. Describe various types of technology used in undergraduate medical education.
5. Discuss uses of technology in undergraduate medical education.

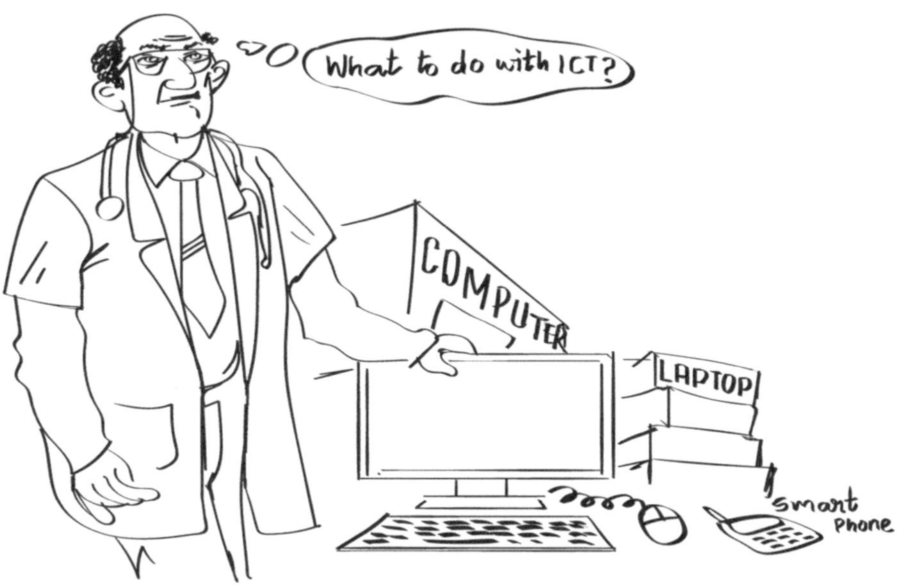

Fig. 5.1 Lack of awareness of the uses of technology

Kadambari D et al., *Improving Discipline-Based Undergraduate Medical Curriculum*, https://doi.org/10.1007/978-981-13-1310-3_5

5.1 Introduction

Use of technology has become a part of our daily life. Technology has also been increasingly used in education including medical education. One advantage of technology is that it can facilitate self-learning. This has been a factor in increasing use of technology in all forms of education. Use of technology is part of global and national recommendations for undergraduate medical education. These include recommendations of Medical Council of India. These recommendations are included in this chapter. Use of technology has advantages and disadvantages which are mentioned. Effectiveness of technology and use of blended learning in undergraduate medical education are described. Various forms of technology such as audiovisual aids, educational media, computers, the Internet, World Wide Web and mobile devices are described in relation to undergraduate medical education. Use of technology in lectures is discussed in detail. Technology can also be used for group discussion, individual learning, assessment and simulation. These uses are described with reference to undergraduate medical education. Learning management system and its uses in education are discussed. Uses of online resources and networking in medical education are also described.

5.2 Global Recommendations for Information and Communication Technology

5.2.1 Global Minimum Essential Requirements in Medical Education

Management of information is one of the seven outcome-competence domains in global minimum essential requirements in medical education (Core Committee, Institute for International Medical Education 2002). The domain of management of information includes the competency of the use of information and communication technology to assist in patient care.

5.2.2 WFME Global Standards

WFME (World Federation for Medical Education) Global Standards for Quality Improvement in Basic Medical Education includes information technology as one of the educational resources (World Federation for Medical Education 2012). As basic standard, the medical school must have a policy for use of information and communication technology in the educational programme. As quality development standard, information and communication technology should be used for accessing information, self-learning and managing patients.

5.3 National Recommendations for Information and Communication Technology

5.3.1 Medical Council of India

Medical Council of India's Regulations on Graduate Medical Education (1997) state in General Considerations and Teaching Approach that 'Integration of ICT in learning process will be implemented'.

Regulations on Graduate Medical Education—Proposed of Medical Council of India (2012)—include lifelong learner committed to continuous improvement of skills and knowledge as one of the five roles for an Indian Medical Graduate. Under the role of lifelong learner includes the competency of 'demonstrate ability to search (including through electronic means), and critically evaluate the medical literature and apply the information in the care of the patient'.

5.3.2 Liaison Committee on Medical Education

According to the Liaison Committee on Medical Education (2016), a medical education programme in the United States and Canada should include opportunities for self-directed learning and independent study to foster the skills necessary for lifelong learning. These skills include information management skills.

5.3.3 General Medical Council

Outcomes for Graduates (*Tomorrow's Doctors*) include the outcome of 'use information effectively in a medical context' under the category of 'The doctor as a practitioner' (General Medical Council (UK) 2015).

5.3.4 Scottish Deans' Medical Education Group

It is one of the twelve domains for The Scottish Doctor Learning Outcomes in medical informatics (Scottish Deans' Medical Education Group 2008). This domain includes accessing data sources and information technology skills.

5.4 Competencies in Information and Communication Technology for Healthcare

The Association of Faculties of Medicine of Canada and Canada Health Infoway (2014) have published eHealth Competencies for Undergraduate Medical Education. They have defined eHealth as 'the appropriate and innovative use of information and communication technologies (ICTs) to enable and improve health and health care services'. These competencies in information and communication technology have been described under the CanMEDS roles. Each competency also includes preclerkship and clerkship milestones. As an example from this competency framework, under the role of a scholar, there is a competency of 'Use information and communication technologies to enhance knowledge, skills and judgement in providing evidence-informed patient care'. Milestones for this competency include learning skills of retrieval and critical appraisal of information from relevant literature in preclerkship phase and improving these skills in clerkship phase (The Association of Faculties of Medicine of Canada and Canada Health Infoway 2014). These eHealth Competencies for Undergraduate Medical Education in a similar fashion also describe competencies and their milestones for the roles of communicator, collaborator, professional, health advocate, medical expert and leader also (The Association of Faculties of Medicine of Canada and Canada Health Infoway 2014). As information and communication technology continues to play an increasing role in daily life, similar changes are likely to occur in provision of healthcare and related information.

5.5 Advantages and Limitations of E-Learning

In the present information age, lifelong learning skills are essential for medical doctors. Thus lifelong learner is one of the five roles described for Indian Medical Graduate (Medical Council of India 2012). This role includes self-directed learning skills which have also been recommended (Medical Council of India 1997, 2012). Information and communication technology is increasingly used for self-directed learning. The government is also promoting self-directed learning using information and communication technology by making available a portal called "Swayam" (2018, https:// swayam.gov.in).

The main advantage of e-learning is that it is controlled by learners (AAMC Institute for Improving Medical Education 2007). This facilitates active learning (McKimm et al. 2003). Learners have liberty to learn anywhere and anytime (AAMC Institute for Improving Medical Education 2007; McKimm et al. 2003). Availability of smartphones has further facilitated learning anywhere and anytime. Learners can pace their learning, and learning can be repeated at any number of times. Thus deliberate practice is possible for skill learning without any harm to patients (AAMC Institute for Improving Medical Education 2007). Individualization of instruction and standardization of instruction and assessment are possible (AAMC Institute for Improving Medical Education 2007). Web-based learning allows linking of resources of different formats (McKimm et al. 2003).

There are also limitations of e-learning. The main limitation is low fidelity and physical interactivity (AAMC Institute for Improving Medical Education 2007). Another limitation is that learners may feel isolated. Without guidance and support, learners may find it difficult to manage e-learning on their own. This is particularly true in situations in which lecture-based teaching is commonly used and self-directed learning is not encouraged in the regular course.

5.6 Effectiveness of E-Learning

As the use of e-learning is increasing in undergraduate medical education, there is a corresponding increase in the research into effectiveness of e-learning. There have been two recent systematic reviews on the impact of e-learning on knowledge, skills, attitudes and satisfaction of undergraduates in health professions (Rasmussen et al. 2014; George et al. 2014). These are briefly described.

Rasmussen et al. (2014) studied the impact of offline e-learning on knowledge, skills, attitudes and satisfaction of undergraduates in health professions. In this systematic review, 49 studies were included, and these involved 4955 students from medical, dentistry, nursing, psychology and physical therapy courses. This systematic review suggested that 'offline e-learning is equivalent and possibly superior to traditional learning regarding knowledge, skills, attitudes and satisfaction'. Authors suggested that offline e-learning can be used in areas having shortage of workforce.

The impact of online e-learning on knowledge, skills, attitudes and satisfaction of undergraduates in health professions was studied by George et al. (2014). In this systematic review, 6750 students from medical, dentistry, nursing, physical therapy and pharmacy courses were involved as part of 59 studies. The results of this systematic review suggested that 'online e-learning is equivalent, possibly superior to traditional learning'.

E-learning is commonly regarded as equivalent to traditional teaching-learning methods. It is seen not as a replacement but as a supplement to traditional methods as part of blended learning (Ruiz et al. 2006). However, e-learning needs to be adopted and integrated into medical education as it provides the advantages of adaptive learning and collaborative learning (Ruiz et al. 2006).

5.7 Blended Learning

Blended learning is a strategy in which e-learning is combined with traditional forms of learning. Theoretically this concept appears to be acceptable, and there are studies also available on blended learning.

Rowe et al. (2012) published a systematic review on the role of blended learning in clinical education of students in health professions. Only seven studies fulfilled inclusion criteria out of 71 articles retrieved. The review only suggested that blended learning has potential to improve clinical competencies of students in healthcare professions. Single studies have also been reported on blended learning (Lipman et al. 2001; Shah et al. 2008; Nkenke et al. 2012; Grasl et al. 2012; Morton et al. 2016). Important points are briefly described from these studies of blended learning. The addition of Internet-based teaching added value to traditional teaching (Lipman et al. 2001). Blended learning is popular with students (Shah et al. 2008). Technology-enhanced learning cannot replace traditional teaching but has potential to reduce the need for lectures (Nkenke et al. 2012). The addition of web-based approach benefitted all students, but students with more previous knowledge were benefited more than students with less previous knowledge (Grasl et al. 2012).

Students liked blended learning 'but only if it was highly structured, of high quality and supported by tutorials' (Morton et al. 2016).

Blended learning including traditional learning and e-learning needs to be used in undergraduate medical education, and both should be integrated for optimum effect.

5.8 Audiovisual Aids

Audiovisual aids are used for oral presentations such as a lecture. These aids include visual aids which can be projected visual aids including PowerPoint slides (using computer and projector) and document camera and non-projected visual aids including chalkboard, whiteboard, interactive whiteboard, charts and cards. Audiovisual aids also include audio aids, e.g. public address system.

5.8.1 PowerPoint Slides Using Computer and Projector

PowerPoint slides are the commonest projected visual aids used for oral presentations. Images of PowerPoint slides from a computer screen are projected on to a projector screen, whiteboard or a white wall using a LCD or DLP projector. Computerless projectors are also available. Modern projectors give visually appealing and high-quality images. These projectors can be place on tables or mounted on ceiling. Projectors with short throw and ultrashort throw are available which can be kept closer to projector screen.

PowerPoint slides can be used for text, graphics and pictures. All material on a PowerPoint slide should be relevant to the objective of the presentation. Legibility of a text slide can be assured by paying attention to the amount of text on a given slide, colours of background and lettering and font. The commonest mistake is to put too much text on a slide, and this can be avoided by following simple guidelines. Commonly, rule of six is recommended in which each slide should have a maximum of six lines and each line should have a maximum of six words. For legibility, colours used for background and lettering should be selected to produce high contrast. One choice is to use white background and a dark colour such as black or blue for lettering. Another choice is to use a dark colour such as blue for background with white lettering. Font type should be a sans-serif variety such as Arial preferably in boldface. Font size should be large enough to be seen clearly from the last row, and in large classes a font size of minimum 30 point may be required. Lower case letters should be preferred as they are easier to read than capital letters. Background of slides along with colour, type and point size of lettering should be consistent in a given presentation.

5.8.2 Document Camera

Document camera is a sophisticated version of overhead projector. Document camera is used with a projector and projection screen. It can directly project images of transparent or opaque objects like an overhead projector. Images of overhead transparencies can be projected. Images of printed and written materials can also be projected. Document camera can also project images of three-dimensional objects such as specimens. A darkened room is not needed, and zooming in and zooming out of objects are possible. An attachment for microscope is also available in some document cameras for projecting microscopic slides.

5.8.3 Chalkboard and Whiteboard

Chalkboard is the most commonly available visual aid which can be made locally. It is also inexpensive, independent of power supply and easy to maintain. Chalkboard is available in various sizes. It permits step by step presentation of concepts. Key words and key messages can be emphasized and explained. It is preferable to use capital letters on chalkboard to maintain uniformity and legibility of writing. Letters should be large enough to be easily read by students in the back rows. Similarly diagrams should also be large enough so they can be easily seen from the back rows. Proper use of chalkboard requires appropriate writing and drawing skills from the teacher. Other limitations include erasing of written matter and drawings which cannot be preserved for future use. Loss of eye contact with students during writing and drawing on chalkboard and pointing at written matter and drawings can be minimized by standing sideways. Effective use of chalkboard requires advance planning for writing and drawing throughout the presentation. Use of whiteboard and whiteboard marking pens can avoid the messiness of the use of chalk pieces.

5.8.4 Interactive Whiteboard

Interactive whiteboard is used in combination with a computer and a digital projector (National Centre for Technology in Education 2009). The computer screen is projected on to the interactive whiteboard. The interactive whiteboard is a special touch-sensitive board which can be operated digitally with a finger or pen (National Centre for Technology in Education 2009). It includes advantages of chalkboard or ordinary whiteboard. In addition any written matter or drawing can be saved in memory for future retrieval. Erase and colour facilities are also included. Work of students can be presented in interactive fashion (National Centre for Technology in Education 2009). Presentation can be enhanced by incorporating still pictures, video and audio to facilitate understanding. Interactive whiteboard is expensive and requires technical support and long learning period, and it needs to be integrated into teaching and learning process (National Centre for Technology in Education 2009). Careful planning is required for effective and efficient use of interactive whiteboard.

5.8.5 Charts and Cards

Flip chart is an effective aid for teaching-learning in small groups. Flash cards can be used for aiding communication in small groups. Both flip charts and flash cards can be used for step by step presentation of material for learning. Flash cards can also be used as an inexpensive audience response system in lectures.

5.8.6 Public Address System

Public address system is an audio aid which consists of microphone, amplifier and speakers. It is required for communication in medium and large groups. Public address system reproduces original sound at a higher intensity. Acoustic features of the room/hall and type of public address system determine the quality of reproduced sound. Volume of sound should be sufficient for the sound to be heard in back rows. Collar mike is to be preferred over hand and table mikes as due to fixed distance between mouth and mike the volume of sound is kept constant.

5.9 Educational Media

Educational media are means to convey educational information. These media include audio media, visual media and multimedia.

5.9.1 Audio Media

Audio media denote sound recordings on compact discs (CDs). Examples of audio media can include recording of presentations by experts, discussion by experts and heart sounds including murmurs. Such media can be used for learning in groups and for individual learning.

5.9.2 Visual Media

Visual media include photographs and videos. Photographs of clinical conditions and specimens can be used for group and individual learning. Videos are very effective educational media. Video recording can be done on CDs and digital versatile discs (DVDs). Videos can be used for teaching-learning of various skills including emergency and non-emergency procedural skills, open and endoscopic surgical skills and communication skills. These videos can be used for large group, small group and individual learning.

5.9.3 Multimedia

Multimedia denotes various combinations of text, pictures, graphics, animation, audio and video. Multimedia constitutes powerful media for educational purposes. Multimedia is used with computer and the Internet and is included in computer-assisted and Internet-based learning resources.

5.10 Computers in Education

Computers (desktops, laptops, tablets and smartphones) are components of information and communication technology and are used for feeding, processing, storing, retrieving and sending information electronically. Computers are widely used in general education and are becoming popular in medical education also. Computers can be used alone and along with the Internet. Offline e-learning (Rasmussen et al. 2014) is an example of isolated use of computers in education. Computers have capability for using multimedia, hyperlinks and searching. Computer-assisted learning and computer-managed learning are two common applications of computers in education.

Computer-assisted learning includes various modes of learning (Narayan and Sethuraman 2000). In drill and practice mode, factual information is learnt by repetition from the material presented in computers. Tutorial mode involves learning in interactive fashion in which feedback is provided to learners for correction and reinforcement. Patient problems can be simulated for learning problem-solving in case-simulation mode. In laboratory mode physiological processes can be simulated in computer programmes, and it can be used for replacing use of animal experimentation. Laboratory simulation mode has been used in pharmacology for learning effects of various drugs (John 2013; Amirtha et al. 2017).

Computer-managed learning is use of computers in managing educational information of students. Learning progress of students can be recorded, and feedback can be provided to them.

5.11 Internet and World Wide Web in Education

The World Wide Web is the largest source of information of various kinds, and it is based on a global computer network, the Internet. The World Wide Web is also the largest information source for medicine and medical education. The Internet and World Wide Web are also the most important systems for communication of information. Computers, the Internet and the World Wide Web are core components of information and communication technology.

E-mail (electronic mail) is a commonly used facility for sending information in the Internet. It is used both for general as well as educational purposes. E-mail can be used for communication of educational information to students, and it can also be used for receiving information from students. Asynchronous discussion using text for collaborative learning can be held among students with moderation by a teacher using e-mail; the Internet is commonly used for online searching of medical literature for patient care and also for research. Institutional website can be used for conveying curricular information to students. Online modules can also be designed for supplementing face-to-face learning in undergraduate medical education as part of a blended learning programme.

Web has evolved from Web 1.0 to Web 2.0. Web 1.0 permitted only reading and downloading. Web 2.0 also permits writing and uploading, creating possibility for participation and interaction. Tools of Web 2.0 are free and easy to use. Blogs and wikis are common Web 2.0 tools. Blogs are like diary pages in which regular entries can be made and the message can reach many readers. Wikis are also Web 2.0 tools which permit content to be entered by members who can also modify and edit the content. Blogs and wikis can be also used in medical education for interactive learning.

5.12 Mobile Devices in Education

The era of mobile technologies started with advent of a handheld personal computer also called personal digital assistant (PDA). Studies have reported about the use of PDAs by undergraduate medical students. In a study reported by Chatterley and Chojecki (2010), common uses of personal digital assistant included calendar, drug reference, e-mail/text and clinical reference text. In another study, uses of personal digital assistant by undergraduate medical students included Dr. Companion (including Oxford Handbook of Clinical Medicine) and other online medical resources (Davies et al. 2012).

Smartphone was the next mobile device which came into popular use. Mosa et al. (2012) published a systematic review of use of smartphones for applications in healthcare. In this study, medical applications for medical and nursing students were described. These applications included various anatomy tools such as Netter's *Atlas of Human Anatomy* with Netter's *Anatomy Flash Cards* (Mosa et al. 2012). Other applications included *Oxford Handbook of Clinical Specialties* (including 12 books) and Mobipocket Reader (an electronic book reader) (Mosa et al. 2012). In addition, applications for healthcare professionals were also used by medical and nursing students for educational purposes. Applications for healthcare professionals included disease diagnosis, drug reference, medical calculators and literature search (Mosa et al. 2012).

Ellaway et al. (2014) did a survey study of undergraduate medical students on their use and attitude towards mobile technology. The study included students from all 4 years of the programme. Mobile devices were defined as cell phones and mobile phones, smartphones and tablets. Medical students were given a laptop and an iPad at the beginning of first year and a laptop and an iPhone at the beginning of third year. Mobile device was found to be very useful in clinical context mostly for personal learning. It was used more for personal learning than for learning in classroom. Thus students adapted the use of mobile devices according to the context. The study of Payne et al. (2012) suggested that ownership of smartphone and its use are high among undergraduate medical students and junior doctors. In another study of attitudes of medical students, residents and teachers towards the use of smartphone (Wallace et al. 2012), the need for policy regarding the use of mobile devices was stressed to benefit from this technology and to avoid any undesirable effects.

It is encouraging to note that there are some studies on the use of mobile devices among medical students from India. In one study by Subba et al. (2013), it was noted that 335 out of 336 medical students owned mobile phones. Most commonly mobile phone was used to talk to parents and friends. Ringxiety or phantom ringing was experienced by nearly one-third of students. Authors noted that students with ringxiety were more likely to use mobile phone in restricted places like classroom and library and reported hampered studies. Authors suggested the need to take appropriate measures for these problems. Subhash and Bapurao (2015) in their study of undergraduate medical students found that most of students had some type of mobile device and they commonly used it for communication, learning and entertainment purposes. The students noted that small screen, lack of time and lack of institutional support are important barriers in the use of mobile phone in education. Most of students wanted some restriction in their use, some wanted a lot of restriction in their use and a smaller number wanted no restriction in their use. The authors suggested that the use of mobile devices should be considered for possible inclusion in undergraduate medical curriculum for learning in view of their increasing use by students.

5.13 Technology for Lectures

Lecture is a commonly used teaching-learning method for large groups. Some form of technology is almost always used in lectures. This technology includes public address system, chalkboard, PowerPoint slides, audience response system, interactive whiteboard and smart classroom, podcasting, technology for flipping the classroom and social media.

5.13.1 Chalkboard

It is interesting to note that there are studies comparing the use of chalkboard with that of PowerPoint published recently from India (de Sa and Keny 2014; Swati et al. 2014; Prabhu et al. 2014; Petimani and Adake 2015; Seth et al. 2010; Jadhav et al. 2016). These studies indicate that chalkboard continues to be used in lectures. Hence it is necessary to use chalkboard effectively keeping in mind necessary measures described earlier.

5.13.2 PowerPoint Slides

For any presentation using PowerPoint, the presentation should be planned first and then only PowerPoint slides should be incorporated as required (Harden 2008). It should not be that PowerPoint slides are made first then the presentation is planned. This concept applies to lectures using PowerPoint slides also. Important measures for making effective PowerPoint slides have been already described earlier. Recently published studies from India comparing the use of PowerPoint with the use of chalkboard in lectures give an indication of the current situation about the use of PowerPoint slides in lectures in India (de Sa and Keny 2014; Swati et al. 2014; Prabhu et al. 2014; Petimani and Adake 2015; Seth et al. 2010; Jadhav et al. 2016). There is a need to emphasize that PowerPoint slides should be used effectively in lectures.

5.13.3 Audience Response System

Audience response system is a device which can elicit responses from all students in a lecture. A simple audience response system consists of the use of coloured flash cards (Teaching with Technology 2007a). Thus four flash cards of different colours can be used to denote four alternatives of a multiple choice question. Students can use these cards to show their responses to a multiple choice question asked by the teacher.

Electronic audience response systems are also called classroom response systems (Teaching with Technology 2007a). Classroom response system consists of a software which can be integrated with the Microsoft PowerPoint in the laptop of the teacher and remote transmitters (clickers) of students (Teaching with Technology 2007a). The teacher can prepare question slides having appropriate questions of true/false type or multiple choice type. Students enter their responses in their remote transmitters. The software in the teacher's laptop converts these responses into tables or graphs which can be immediately displayed in the PowerPoint slide. Classroom response system software can also permit the teacher to transfer and save data for further analysis. Classroom response system can also be integrated with learning management systems. Responses of students can be used for initiating peer discussion and clarification of concepts.

A systematic review of the effects of audience response systems in health professions education has been published by Nelson et al. (2012). This review included analysis of 21 studies. Twenty studies pertained to the use of audience response system in lectures, and 14 studies involved undergraduate students. This systematic review suggested that audience response system can create interactive environment and may improve knowledge scores. While using audience response system in lectures, some important points to be followed are that proper planning and rehearsal of the presentation should be done and students should be prepared for the session (Robertson 2000). Questions should be asked for only important concepts, and they should be kept simple.

5.13.4 Interactive Whiteboard and Smart Classroom

Interactive whiteboard is an advanced technology which can integrate various educational resources in the classroom for interactive learning. Interactive whiteboard along with audience response system and automatic recording system are key components of a smart classroom (Tai et al. 2017). Smart classroom facilitates learner-centred teaching.

5.13.5 Podcasting

Recording of lectures is done so these recordings can be used by students for review and revision. The recording can be in audio or video mode. As lectures are regularly held in a programme, it will be useful if students can receive audio/video recordings of lectures on a regular basis. This has become possible with podcasting. Podcasting includes not only publishing of a series of audio/video content on the web but also permits people to subscribe to and receive the series in an automatic way (Teaching with Technology 2007b). Seamless dissemination of audio or video content to people or sites that have chosen to receive it is made possible by RSS (Real Simple Syndication) feed (also called a stream). An Aggregator is a software which gathers RSS feeds from various websites and delivers them in an easy-to-read format to receiving people or websites. Podcasting permits students to receive recorded lectures from various websites (Teaching with Technology 2007b). Podcasting method increases the chances that students will download the files, and audio recording was preferred format for lectures (Teaching with Technology 2007b). Studies have shown that podcasting has little effect on attendance in lectures (Teaching with Technology 2007b).

5.13.6 Technology for Flipping the Classroom

The flipped classroom is an educational approach in which the usual sequence of lecture and homework are reversed (Moffett 2015). Initial homework preparation is used to address lower cognitive levels of learning, and lecture time is devoted to higher cognitive levels of learning (Moffett 2015). Initial preparation activities can include print-, audio- or video-based material (Sharma et al. 2015). Podcasts can also be used for initial preparation (Moffett 2015). Audience response system is necessary for interactive learning during lecture time.

5.13.7 Social Media

Social media are popular among medical students. Thus it is natural that these may be used for enhancing learning during lectures. George et al. (2013) published a study in which Google Docs and SurveyMonkey were used during lectures. Lectures were part of a course for first year medical students. Google Docs enabled students to anonymously ask questions, and SurveyMonkey allowed students to respond to survey questions. Careful preparation was done to integrate the use of Google Docs and SurveyMonkey in the lectures. This use of social media facilitated interaction between teacher and students and among students (George et al. 2013). It also gave students some control over content and flow of lectures (George et al. 2013). The authors recommended the integration of social media into the course. They also stated that the media cannot replace accepted active educational approaches of case-based learning, problem-based learning and team-based learning. However, social media can be used to complement active learning methods.

5.14 Technology for Group Discussion

Group discussion is a useful method which uses active learning and collaborative learning principles. It needs moderation skills of teachers, and students should be prepared for the discussion method. It is possible to use technology for group discussion. Online discussion can be synchronous or asynchronous. Synchronous group discussion can be done using audio and video conferencing. In web conferencing web cameras and computers are used for carrying out discussion. Synchronous online discussion can also be done using bulletin boards and chatrooms. Asynchronous online discussion is usually done using e-mail. Care should be taken to plan properly any use of online discussion for MBBS students, and learning objectives should initiate the planning. Online discussion sessions should be integrated in the curriculum to make them effective.

5.15 Technology for Individual Learning

Present-day undergraduate medical students have adequate skills to use computer, the Internet and smartphone. They are already using these technological devices for their individual learning. It is time for us to acknowledge this fact and judiciously incorporate the use of these devices in undergraduate medical education so that medical students learn to use these devices effectively under the guidance and support of their teachers.

5.16 Technology for Assessment

Technology is already being used in entrance tests for undergraduate medical education. These tests are based on multiple choice questions. These tests are administered online. The other advantage is that scoring is automated. It is also possible to do item analysis using software, and item banks can be created. Computer-based testing using multiple choice questions can also be used for summative assessments. Formative assessment can also be done using technology in lecture setting. Three to five multiple choice questions can be used for assessing main points towards the end of a lecture using PowerPoint technology and audience response system. This simple method needs to be utilized on a regular basis in order to make formative assessments an integral part of undergraduate medical educational programmes.

5.17 Technology for Simulation

After the publication of *To Err is Human: Building a Safer Health System* (Kohn et al. 1999), patient safety has become an essential component of undergraduate medical curriculum. The third level of Miller's pyramid ('Shows how') concerns the use of simulation (Miller 1990). The use of simulation obviates any harm to patients and allows repeated practice by students. A list of essential skills for undergraduate medical education in the Indian context was published in the mid-1990s (Sethuraman and Kumar 1996). This list included both emergency and non-emergency skills. Technology available for learning these skills includes partial-task trainers, patient simulators and screen-based simulators. Partial-task trainers are used for learning procedural skills such as nasogastric intubation and urinary bladder catheterization. Patient simulators can simulate physiological features and certain clinical conditions. Patient simulators are placed in a simulated environment (e.g. emergency room) for facilitating learning of the management of given clinical conditions. Screen-based simulators produce clinical scenarios on a computer screen. Students can interact with the virtual patient to learn about history taking, physical examination, diagnosis and management of the given problem. Screen-based virtual reality simulation can enable learning of surgical procedures such as cystoscopy.

5.18 Learning Management Systems

Information management systems are commonly used in medical institutions for management of hospital- and administration-related information. Similarly, learning management systems are used in education by educational institutions. A learning management system may contain information related to curriculum, outcome-competencies, course content, teaching-learning activities and assessment of educational outcomes. This will enable educational management to track learning progress of all students. Learning management system can also contain personal particulars and attendance details of all students. Teaching-learning activities may include collaborative tools such as discussion boards. Learning management system can include assessment tools and storage of assessment information. Learning management system can provide links to the World Wide Web also. For optimum usefulness, the learning management system should be integrated with face-to-face learning programme for a given educational programme as part of blended learning.

5.19 Online Resources in Medical Education

In spite of the pioneering role of National Teacher Training Centres and commendable efforts of Medical Education Units and Medical Council of India's Basic Courses in Medical Education Technologies, the undergraduate medical education in India remains variable and needs to be improved. The last major revision of undergraduate medical curriculum was done in 1997. In fact there is a view that the *Flexner Report* published in 1910 in the United States is relevant to medical education in South Asia including India (Amin et al. 2010). Efforts need to be directed towards implementation of national guidelines in undergraduate medical education. Side-by-side relevant research in medical education needs also to be done.

In view of the foregoing, we need to become aware of medical education literature for improving education and research in undergraduate medical education. For this purpose, we need to be familiar with important online resources in medical education.

Articles on medical education are published from time to time in all general and speciality medical journals. Common journals which are totally devoted to medical education include *Medical Teacher*, *Academic Medicine*, *Medical Education*, *Clinical Teacher*, *BMC Medical Education*, *Advances in Health Sciences Education: Theory and Practice*, *Teaching and Learning in Medicine*, *Education for Health* and *Journal of Graduate Medical Education*. All these journals are available in online versions.

5.20 Technology for Networking

There are a number of medical colleges in India situated in different geographical regions of the country. In relation to undergraduate medical education, faculty in different medical colleges are likely to have expertise in different areas of education such as curriculum, objectives, teaching-learning, assessment and governance. If appropriate consortia are formed for different educational areas by faculty of different colleges, the expertise can be pooled and used for mutual benefit of all medical colleges.

Our country is diverse and different ailments and diseases may be prevalent in different areas of the country. Consequent to centralized admission policy for undergraduate medical education, many students study in some parts of the country and later practise in other parts of the country. As some ailments and diseases are common but others are different, a particular student may not be able to get the total picture of patient problems. To enable all students to get a reasonable holistic picture of patient problems, consortia of faculty from different medical colleges can be used to make video presentations of those clinical cases which are likely to be different among medical colleges. These video recordings can be made available in all medical colleges so all medical students in the country can benefit and have a holistic picture of patient problems.

Information and communication technology can be used during various stages of developing common resources for undergraduate medical education. Later these resources can be made available on a suitable online platform so they can be used by medical faculty and students in all medical colleges.

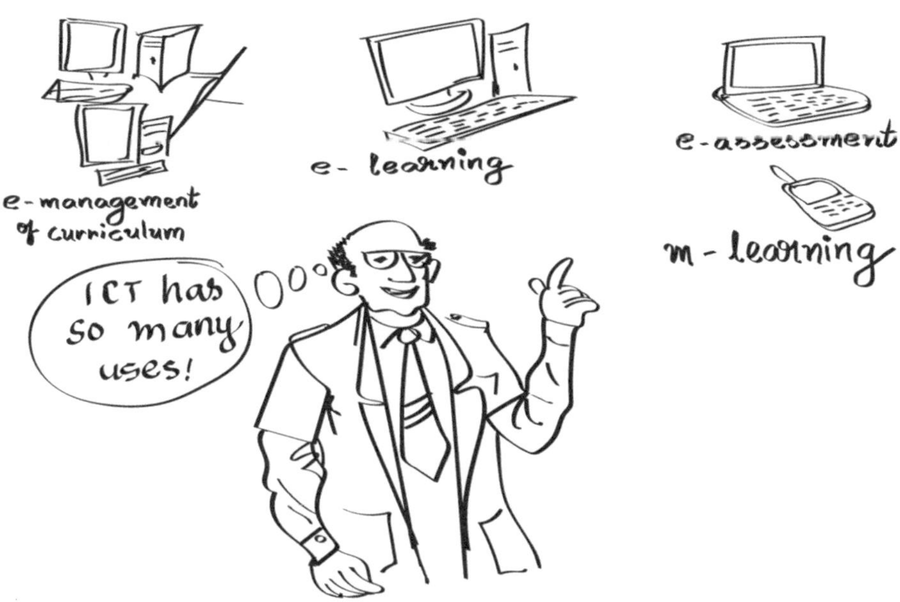

Fig. 5.2 Awareness about multiple uses of technology

Conclusions

Use of technology is a part of various global and national recommendations for undergraduate medical education. Medical Council of India has also recommended the use of technology in undergraduate medical education. One advantage of technology is that it facilitates self-learning. Technology should be used as a part of blended learning. Technology can be used in various steps of undergraduate medical education. Use of technology must be integrated in undergraduate medical curriculum for its effectiveness.

References

AAMC Institute for Improving Medical Education (2007) Effective use of educational technology in medical education. Association of American Medical Colleges, Mar 2007. Available from https://members.aamc.org/eweb/upload/Effective%20Use%20of%20Educational.pdf. Accessed 12 Jan 2018

Amin Z, Burdick WP, Supe A, Singh T (2010) Relevance of the Flexner report to contemporary medical education in South Asia. Acad Med 85(2):333–339. https://doi.org/10.1097/ACM.0b013e3181c874cb

Amirtha R, Gupta R, Rehan HS, Gupta LK (2017) Impact of computer assisted learning as teaching modality on learning and understanding of pharmacology among undergraduate medical students. Indian J Physiol Pharmacol 61(2):202–207 Available from https://pdfs.semanticscholar.org/2ad9/761a3f681e8ea75554f6d27b2c79044f8564.pdf. Accessed 12 Jan 2018

Chatterley T, Chojecki D (2010) Personal digital assistant usage among undergraduate medical students: exploring trends, barriers, and the advent of smartphones. J Med Libr Assoc 98(2):157–160. PMCID: PMC2859274. https://doi.org/10.3163/1536-5050.98.2.008

Core Committee, Institute for International Medical Education (2002) Global minimum essential requirements in medical education. Med Teach 24(2):130–135. PMID: 12098431. https://doi.org/10.1080/01421590220120731

Davies BS, Rafique J, Vincent TR, Fairclough J, Packer MH, Vincent R et al (2012) Mobile medical education (MoMed) – how mobile information resources contribute to learning for undergraduate clinical students – a mixed methods study. BMC Med Educ 12:1. https://doi.org/10.1186/1472-6920-12-1

Ellaway RH, Fink P, Graves L, Campbell A (2014) Left to their own devices: medical learners' use of mobile technologies. Med Teach 36(2):130–138. PMID: 24195445. https://doi.org/10.3109/0142159X.2013.849800

General Medical Council (2015) Outcomes for graduates (Tomorrow's Doctors), July 2015. Available from https://www.gmc-uk.org/Outcomes_for_graduates_Jul_15_1216.pdf_61408029.pdf. Accessed 8 Jan 2018

George DR, Dreibelbis TD, Aumiller B (2013) How we used two social media tools to enhance aspects of active learning during lectures. Med Teach 35:985–988. PMID: 23902318. https://doi.org/10.3109/0142159X.2013.818631

George PP, Papachristou N, Belisario JM, Wang W, Wark PA, Cotic Z et al (2014) Online eLearning for undergraduates in health professions: a systematic review of the impact on knowledge, skills, attitudes and satisfaction. J Glob Health 4(1):010406. PMCID: PMC4073252. https://doi.org/10.7189/jogh.04.010406

Grasl MC, Pokieser P, Gleiss A, Brandstaetter J, Sigmund T, Erovic BM et al (2012) A new blended learning concept for medical students in otolaryngology. Arch Otolaryngol Head Neck Surg 138(4):358–365 Available from https://pdfs.semanticscholar.org/f4f2/087134620abd7696255ef1f31a555a4201ce.pdf. Accessed 12 Jan 2018

Harden RM (2008) Death by PowerPoint – the need for a 'fidget index'. Med Teach 30:833–835. PMID: 19117220. https://doi.org/10.1080/01421590802307743

Jadhav VS, Adchitre SA, Magare AR, Surve RR, Mahajan SM (2016) A comparative study of blackboard teaching with PowerPoint teaching in third year medical students. Int J Curr Med Appl Sci 11(1):17–21 Available from www.ijcmaas.com/pdffileDownload?id=362. Accessed 12 Jan 2018

John LJ (2013) A review of computer assisted learning in medical undergraduates. J Pharmacol Pharmacother 4(2):86–90. PMCID: PMC3669587. https://doi.org/10.4103/0976-500X.110870

Kohn L, Corrigan J, Donaldson M (1999) To err is human: building a safer health system. National Academy Press, Washington, DC

Liaison Committee on Medical Education 2016 Functions and structure of a medical school. Standards for accreditation of medical education programs leading to the M.D. degree, Mar 2016. Available from https://med.virginia.edu/ume-curriculum/wp-content/uploads/sites/216/2016/07/2017-18_Functions-and-Structure_2016-03-24.pdf. Accessed 12 Jan 2018

Lipman AJ, Sade RM, Glotzbach AL, Lancaster CJ, Marshall MF (2001) The incremental value of internet-based instruction as an adjunct to classroom instruction: a prospective randomized study. Acad Med 76(10):1060–1064 PMID: 11597850

McKimm J, Jollie C, Cantillon P (2003) Web based learning. In: Cantillon P, Hutchinson L, Wood D (eds) ABC of learning and teaching in medicine, 1st edn. BMJ Publishing Group Ltd., London, pp 42–45

Medical Council of India (1997) Regulations on graduate medical education. Available from https://www.mciindia.org/documents/rulesAndRegulations/GME_REGULA TIONS.pdf. Accessed 8 Jan 2018

Medical Council of India (2012) Regulations on graduate medical education – proposed. Available from http://iafmonline.in/data/circular-notifications/Revised-GME-2012.pdf. Accessed 8 Jan 2018

Miller GE (1990) The assessment of clinical skills/competence/performance. Acad Med 65(Suppl 9):S63–S67 Available from http://winbev.pbworks.com/f/Assessment.pdf. Accessed 12 Jan 2018

Moffett J (2015) Twelve tips for "flipping" the classroom. Med Teach 37:331–336. https://doi.org/10.3109/0142159X.2014.943710

Morton CE, Saleh SN, Smith SF, Hemani A, Ameen A, Bennie TD et al (2016) Blended learning: how can we optimise undergraduate student engagement? BMC Med Educ 16:195. PMID: 27492157. PMCID: PMC4973547. https://doi.org/10.1186/s12909-016-0716-z

Mosa ASM, Yoo J, Sheets L (2012) A systematic review of healthcare applications for smartphones. BMC Med Inform Decis Mak 12:67. PMID: 22781312. PMCID: PMC3534499. https://doi.org/10.1186/1472-6947-12-67

Narayan KA, Sethuraman KR (2000) Computer assisted learning. In: Ananthakrishnan N, Sethuraman KR, Kumar S (eds) Medical education: principles and practice, 2nd edn. National Teacher Training Centre, JIPMER, Pondicherry, pp 73–78

National Centre for Technology in Education (2009) NCTE advice sheet-interactive whiteboards. Advice sheet 16, Nov 2009. Available from http://www.pdsttechnologyineducation.ie/en/Technology/Advice-Sheets/Interactive-Whiteboards.pdf. Accessed 12 Jan 2018

Nelson C, Hartling L, Campbell S, Oswald AE (2012) The effects of audience response systems on learning outcomes in health professions education. A BEME systematic review: BEME Guide No. 21. Med Teach 34(6):e386–e405. PMID: 22578049. https://doi.org/10.3109/0142159X.2012.680938

Nkenke E, Vairaktaris E, Bauersachs A, Eitner S, Budach A, Knipfer C et al (2012) Acceptance of technology-enhanced learning for a theoretical radiological science course: a randomized controlled trial. BMC Med Educ 12:18. PMCID: PMC3353831. https://doi.org/10.1186/1472-6920-12-18

Payne KFB, Wharrad H, Watts K (2012) Smartphone and medical related App use among medical students and junior doctors in the United Kingdom (UK): a regional survey. BMC Med Inform Decis Mak 12:121. PMID: 23110712. PMCID: PMC3504572. https://doi.org/10.1186/1472-6947-12-121

Petimani MS, Adake P (2015) Blackboard versus PowerPoint presentation: students opinion in medical education. Int J Educ Psychol Res 1:289–292. https://doi.org/10.4103/2395-2296.163935 Available from http://www.ijeprjournal.org/temp/IntJEducPsycholRes14289-5000712_012320.pdf. Accessed 12 Jan 2018

Prabhu R, Pai KM, Prabhu G, Shrilatha (2014) A lecture in medical physiology – PowerPoint versus chalkboard. South East Asian J Med Educ 8(1):72–76 Available from http://imsear.li.mahidol.ac.th/bitstream/123456789/166195/1/seajme2014v8n1p72.pdf. Accessed 12 Jan 2018

Rasmussen K, Belisario JM, Wark PA, Molina JA, Loong SL, Cotic Z et al (2014) Offline eLearning for undergraduates in health professions: a systematic review of the impact on knowledge, skills, attitudes and satisfaction. J Glob Health 4(1):010405. https://doi.org/10.7189/jogh.04.010405

Robertson LJ (2000) Twelve tips for using a computerized interactive audience response system. Med Teach 22(3):237–239. https://doi.org/10.1080/01421590050006179

Rowe M, Frantz J, Bozalek V (2012) The role of blended learning in the clinical education of healthcare students: a systematic review. Med Teach 34(4):e216–e221. PMID: 22455712. https://doi.org/10.3109/0142159X.2012.642831

Ruiz JG, Mintzer MJ, Leipzig RM (2006) The impact of E-learning in medical education. Acad Med 81(3):207–212 PMID: 16501260

de Sa SB, Keny MS (2014) PowerPoint versus chalkboard based lectures in pharmacology: evaluation of their impact on medical student's knowledge and their preferences. Int J Adv Health Sci 1(5):10–14 Available from http://www.ijahs.net/uploads/2/6/7/7/26772457/ijahs_vol_1_issue_5_2.pdf. Accessed 12 Jan 2018

Scottish Dean's Medical Education Group (2008) The Scottish Doctor: learning outcomes for the medical undergraduate in Scotland: a foundation for competent and reflective practitioners,

3rd edn. Association for Medical Education in Europe (AMEE), Dundee Available from http://www.scottishdoctor.org/resources/scotdoc3.pdf. Accessed 8 Jan 2018
Seth V, Upadhyaya P, Ahmad M, Moghe V (2010) PowerPoint or chalk and talk: perceptions of medical students versus dental students in a medical college in India. Adv Med Educ Pract 1:11–16. https://doi.org/10.2147/AMEP.S12154
Sethuraman KR, Kumar S (1996) Implementing innovations in clinical skills training (proceedings of a workshop). National Teacher Training Centre, JIPMER, Pondicherry
Shah IM, Walters MR, McKillop JH (2008) Acute medicine teaching in an undergraduate medical curriculum: a blended learning approach. Emerg Med J 25(6):354–357. PMID: 18499818. https://doi.org/10.1136/emj.2007.053082
Sharma N, Lau CS, Doherty I, Harbutt D (2015) How we flipped the medical classroom. Med Teach 37:327–330. PMID: 24934251. https://doi.org/10.3109/0142159X.2014.923821
Subba SH, Mandelia C, Pathak V, Reddy D, Goel A, Tayal A et al (2013) Ringxiety and the mobile phone usage pattern among the students of a medical college in South India. J Clin Diagn Res 7(2):205–209. PMCID: PMC3592275. https://doi.org/10.7860/JCDR/2013/4652.2729
Subhash TS, Bapurao TS (2015) Perception of medical students for utility of mobile technology use in medical education. Int J Med Pub Health 5:305–311. https://doi.org/10.4103/2230-8598.165959
Swati SMC, Suresh SRT, Sachin SGD (2014) Student assessment on learning based on PowerPoint versus chalkboard. Int J Recent Trends Sci Technol 13(2):347–351 Available from http://www.statperson.com/Journal/ScienceAndTechnology/Article/Volume13Issue2/13_2_30.pdf. Accessed 12 Jan 2018
Swayam (2018) Available from https://swayam.gov.in/About. Accessed 12 Jan 2018
Tai Y, Wushuo Y, Kun S (2017) Explore the medical curriculum teaching development in the smart classroom. Int J Inf Educ Technol 7(2):130–134. https://doi.org/10.18178/ijiet.2017.7.2.854
Teaching with Technology (2007a) Classroom response systems. A teaching with technology white paper, Nov 2007. Available from https://www.cmu.edu/teaching/technology/whitepapers/ClassroomResponse_Nov07.pdf. Accessed 12 Jan 2018
Teaching with Technology (2007b) Podcasting. A teaching with technology white paper, June 2007. Available from https://www.cmu.edu/teaching/technology/whitepapers/Podcasting_Jun07.pdf. Accessed 12 Jan 2018
The Association of Faculties of Medicine of Canada and Canada Health Infoway (2014) eHealth competencies for undergraduate medical education. The Association of Faculties of Medicine of Canada, May 2014. Available from https://chec-cesc.afmc.ca/en/system/files/documents/ehealth-competencies-ume_en.pdf. Accessed 12 Jan2018
Wallace S, Clark M, White J (2012) "'It's on my iPhone": attitudes to the use of mobile computing devices in medical education, a mixed-methods study. BMJ Open 2:e001099. https://doi.org/10.1136/bmjopen-2012-001099
World Federation for Medical Education (2012) Basic medical education. WFME Global Standards for quality improvement. The 2012 revision. WFME, Copenhagen Available from http://www.um.es/documents/1935287/1936044/Revision_of_Standards_ for_Basic_Medical_Education_FINAL_260912.pdf/5866f7af-f7fc-4f9a-a7e6-eb054b7795c3. Accessed 8 Jan 2018

Developing Soft Skills

6

Objectives

1. List global and national recommendations for developing soft skills in undergraduate medical curriculum.
2. Describe soft skills which are essential in undergraduate medical education.
3. Discuss methods for developing soft skills in medical students.

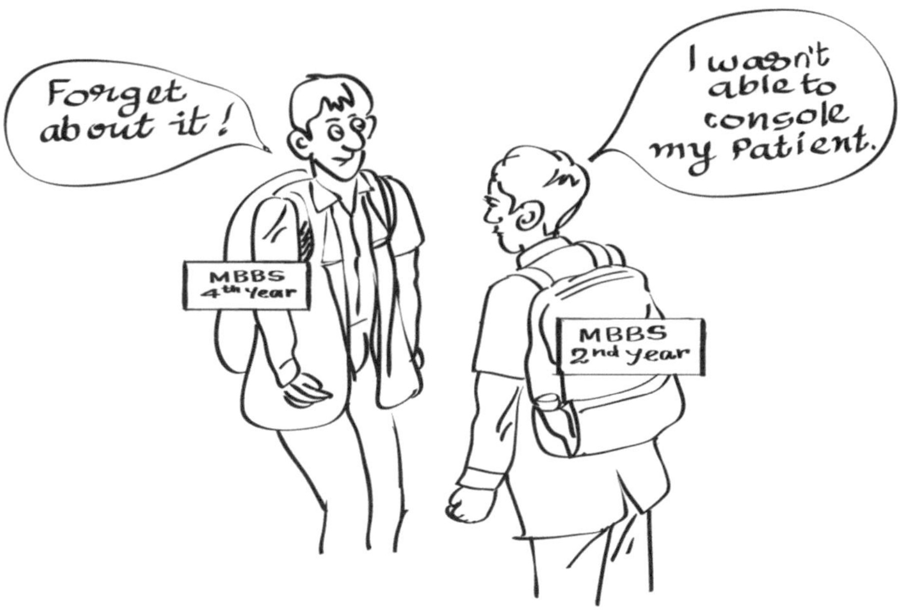

Fig. 6.1 Ignoring soft skills

Kadambari D et al., *Improving Discipline-Based Undergraduate Medical Curriculum*, https://doi.org/10.1007/978-981-13-1310-3_6

6.1 Introduction

Soft skills are necessary for effective functioning of medical doctors. These soft skills include communication skills, teamwork skills and leadership and professionalism. It is important to include methods for developing these skills in undergraduate medical curriculum. There are global recommendations and national recommendations including recommendations of Medical Council of India for developing soft skills in undergraduate medical education. These recommendations are briefly described. Communication skills are essential component of modern undergraduate medical curriculum. Types of communication include oral communication and written communication in different settings. Methods for developing communication skills in undergraduate medical curriculum are mentioned. Teamwork skills can be developed by group discussion, team-based learning and interprofessional education. Opportunities available for developing leadership skills in medical students are listed. Various methods important for developing professionalism in medical students are discussed. Longitudinal courses are essential for developing soft skills in undergraduate medical students. Longitudinal courses used and suggested for medical students in India are described.

6.2 Soft Skills in Undergraduate Medical Education

> Harmonious development of the head, hand and heart is the mark of a model man.
>
> Swami Vivekananda

Effective functioning of a medical doctor requires a balanced combination of knowledge, skills and attitudes. In a traditional discipline-based undergraduate medical curriculum, there is more emphasis on knowledge and skills and less emphasis on attitudes. Attitudes form a key component of soft skills. Soft skills for undergraduate medical curriculum have included communication skills, interpersonal and social skills and professional and ethical attitudes (Van Staden et al. 2006). Common soft skills needed for medical doctors include communication skills, teamwork skills and leadership and professionalism. These soft skills are included in the three of five roles of the Indian Medical Graduate in Regulations on Graduate Medical Education—Proposed of Medical Council of India (2012) and in the four of seven roles of medical doctors in *CanMEDS 2015 Physician Competency Framework* (Frank et al. 2015). Integration of measures for developing soft skills in undergraduate medical educational programme is essential for holistic development of medical students.

6.3 Global Recommendations for Developing Soft Skills

6.3.1 Global Minimum Essential Requirements in Medical Education

Global minimum essential requirements in medical education (Core Committee, Institute for International Medical Education 2002) includes seven outcome-competence domains of which three domains pertain to soft skills. The domain of professional values, attitudes, behaviour and ethics includes 11 competencies. Teamwork skills and leadership are included in the domain of population health and health systems. The domain of communication skills includes nine competencies.

6.3.2 WFME Global Standards

Various outcomes pertaining to soft skills are included as basic standard in WFME (World Federation for Medical Education) Global Standards for Quality Improvement in Basic Medical Education (World Federation for Medical Education 2012). These outcomes include the roles of communicator, manager and professional for medical doctors. Relevant portions of medical ethics, medical jurisprudence and human rights are also included. A proper conduct of students must be ensured by the use of a written code of conduct.

6.4 National Recommendations for Developing Soft Skills

6.4.1 Medical Council of India

One of the five national goals for undergraduate medical education is that at the time of graduation, the medical student will be able to 'become exemplary citizen by observation of medical ethics and fulfilling social and professional obligations, so as to respond to national aspirations' in Medical Council of India's Regulations on Graduate Medical Education (1997). The institutional goals include acquisition of communication skills, ability to work as a leader in healthcare teams, and acquisition of basic management skills pertaining to resource management, general management and hospital management.

Five roles have been included for Indian Medical Graduate in Regulations on Graduate Medical Education— Proposed of Medical Council of India (2012). Of these three roles of communicator, leader and member of the healthcare team and system and professional deal with soft skills. There are four competencies under the role of communicator, six competencies for the role of leader and member of the healthcare team and system and five competencies under the role of professional.

6.4.2 Liaison Committee on Medical Education

The content for educational programme for the M.D. degree in the United States and Canada recommended by Liaison Committee on Medical Education (2016) includes instruction in communication skills, medical ethics and collaborative skills.

6.4.3 General Medical Council

Outcomes for graduates (Tomorrow's Doctors) (General Medical Council (UK) 2015) include the outcome of 'communicate effectively with patients and colleagues in a medical context' under the category of 'The doctor as a practitioner'. The category of 'The doctor as a professional' included the outcomes 'The graduate will be able to behave according to ethical and legal principles' and 'Learn and work effectively within a multiprofessional team'.

6.4.4 Scottish Deans' Medical Education Group

Three of the 12 domains for The Scottish Doctor learning outcomes pertain to soft skills (Scottish Deans' Medical Education Group 2008). The domain of 'communication' has seven outcomes, and the domain of 'attitudes, ethical understanding and legal responsibilities' has nine outcomes. The domain of 'the role of the doctor within the health service' has outcomes of 'The doctor as a manager' and 'The doctor as a member of a multiprofessional team …'.

6.4.5 CanMEDS 2015 Physician Competency Framework

There are seven roles in *CanMEDS 2015 Physician Competency Framework*, and four of these pertain to soft skills (Frank et al. 2015). These include the roles of communicator, collaborator, leader and professional. The role of communicator has five key competencies, the role of collaborator has three, the role of leader has four, and the role of professional has four key competencies. Each of the key competencies includes several enabling competencies.

6.5 Communication Skills

The importance of communication skills is recognized by all, and communication is part of all outcome-competency frameworks. As an example, The Scottish Doctor learning outcomes include communication under three domains (Scottish Deans' Medical Education Group 2008). The domain of clinical skills included history taking. The domain of communication includes general principles of communication and communication with patients and other stakeholders. General principles include oral presentations and writing reports and research papers. The domain of medical informatics includes writing patient records. Communication is a vast area, and only important points in developing communication in undergraduate medical education are briefly described. If active learning methods are used, there will be a lot of opportunities for students to develop good communication skills.

Oral presentations by medical students should be commonly used throughout the undergraduate programme. These presentations can be individual or group presentations. Oral presentations have been used in anatomy as a learning method and also a method to improve speaking skills (Sugand et al. 2010). Use of group discussions in undergraduate programme will also promote active learning and speaking skills. As oral presentations and group discussions are increasingly used in school education, medical students should be comfortable with these methods with proper guidance. It is useful to remember that the use of seminars and group discussions is recommended by Medical Council of India's Regulations on Graduate Medical Education (1997, 2012).

Written assignments are very useful in promoting logical thinking and written communication in English. These assignments should be properly planned and should be returned to students with written feedback by teachers for necessary corrections. In the absence of written assignments, only opportunity for written communication for students may be during summative assessments.

Communication with patients is crucial for good medical care. It is well known that effective doctor-patient communication is associated with better health outcomes, increased satisfaction for both patients and doctors and decreased risk of litigation for doctors (Losh et al. 2005). The Kalamazoo Consensus Statement (Anon 2001) includes seven essential tasks in doctor-patient communication. These include 'build the doctor-patient relationship', 'open the discussion', 'gather information', 'understand the patient's perspective', 'share information', 'reach agreement on problems and plans' and 'provide closure'. Developing skills for these tasks essentially needs repeated practice by students and receiving feedback from teachers. This process can be systematically facilitated by using Miller's pyramid (Miller 1990). 'Knows' level involves knowing about dos and don'ts of doctor-patient communication by reading about relevant case studies. At 'knows how' level, video triggers or live role plays are used to display good and bad examples and initiate group discussions among students. The group discussions are moderated by a teacher. 'Shows how' level involves every student practicing with a role player or a simulated patient. At 'does' level every student interacts with a patient. The teacher provides feedback to students at least two levels. Good and bad examples from real patient records can be used as triggers to initiate group discussions among students with moderation by a teacher for learning about writing proper patient records.

6.6 Teamwork Skills and Leadership

As healthcare delivery needs healthcare teams, the ability to work effectively in healthcare teams is an important soft skill for healthcare professionals including medical doctors. Teamwork skills are combined with leadership in a single role in the roles of Indian Medical Graduate in Regulations on Graduate Medical

Education—Proposed of Medical Council of India (2012). However, in *CanMEDS 2015 Physician Competency Framework* (Frank et al. 2015), teamwork skills come under the role of collaborator, and the role of leader is separate. Teamwork skills can be developed through group discussion method, team-based learning and interprofessional education.

Group discussion is an active learning method which involves discussion among students with teacher being the moderator. It is a small group teaching-learning method involving up to 30 students. However, for optimum discussion, the maximum number of students should be 10. It is a structured learning method with definite predefined objectives and advance planning. Well conducted group discussion can facilitate teamwork and promote learning with understanding. A major limitation of group discussion is the need to have adequate spaces, required number of teachers and enough time.

Team-based learning (Parmelee et al. 2013) is an active learning method which overcomes the limitations of group discussion mentioned earlier. Team-based learning can be held in a lecture hall with single teacher using small groups of students. Common steps of team-based learning include 'advance assignment', 'individual readiness assurance test', 'team readiness assurance test', 'instructor clarification review', 'team application' and 'appeal' (Parmelee et al. 2013). Assignment is done before class and other five steps are done during the class. In assignment, students are given learning objectives and learning materials. Individual readiness is tested by answering multiple choice questions. Team readiness is tested by answering same multiple choice questions using consensus arrived through discussion. Immediate feedback on answers is provided. This may require the use of audience response system. In the next step, the instructor provides clarification for difficult concepts to students. In team application step students are given a scenario involving an important problem. The teams have to discuss the scenario and choose from a range of options. Selected options are made known to the entire class. Individual teams may have to argue for their selected options. All teams are given the same problem (Parmelee et al. 2013). In the step of appeal, a team may suggest an alternative to the option selected by the instructor with supporting evidence (Parmelee et al. 2013). Team-based learning can facilitate understanding of concepts and their use for solving problems. Team-based learning also promotes teamwork. Team-based learning has been used in anatomy teaching-learning. Vasan et al. (2008) replaced most of the lectures for teaching gross anatomy and embryology by team-based learning. They stated that team-based learning was associated with active learning and improved performance of students.

Interprofessional education (IPE) occurs 'when students from two or more professions learn about, from and with each other to enable effective collaboration and improve health outcomes' (World Health Organization 2010). The Lancet Commission report 'Health Professionals for a New Century: Transforming Education to Strengthen Health Systems in an Interdependent World' included interprofessional and transprofessional education as an instructional reform (Frenk et al. 2010). Interprofessional education promotes collaborative practice and better health outcomes (World Health Organization 2010). Interprofessional education has been used in teaching-learning of gross anatomy (Hamilton et al. 2008). Students from various health professions can be involved in interprofessional education during clinical postings (Thistlethwaite 2013). Interprofessional education should be integrated in the undergraduate medical curriculum for optimum benefit.

Leadership opportunities for medical students are usually restricted to organization of cultural programmes. However, it is possible to integrate leadership activities in undergraduate curriculum. Organization of service events as part of service learning can be done by students (Gliatto and Stern 2013). Students can also lead in organization of support activities for their peers. Team-based learning can also provide leadership opportunities. Team-based learning can be used throughout undergraduate medical curriculum. Group assignments and group projects also include leadership opportunities.

6.7 Professionalism

Professionalism denotes 'the competence or skill expected of a professional' (Concise Oxford English Dictionary 2004). Professionalism in medicine includes general responsibilities of a physician. There is a widely accepted charter on professionalism in medicine (Anon 2002). This charter includes three principles and ten professional commitments. Indian Medical Council (2002) has published Professional Conduct, Etiquette and Ethics Regulations. These regulations include a code of medical ethics and duties of physicians to their patients, in consultation, to each other and to the public and to the paramedical profession. Some parts of professionalism such as medical ethics and consent have been part of the course of medical jurisprudence. However, it has been a practice in the United States (Miles et al. 1989) and other countries to have separate courses on ethics and professionalism. Separate course on medical ethics has also been reported from India (Ravindran et al. 1997). The need to have separate courses on ethics and professionalism has arisen because the traditional method of apprenticeship is no longer considered to be enough to develop professionalism.

Formal courses, role modelling and reflection and service learning are three approaches which have been suggested for developing professionalism (Gliatto and Stern 2013). Teaching methods which are employed in formal courses can include interactive presentations, group discussions and role plays. Trigger films can be used to initiate discussion (Ber and Alroy 2002). Role modelling is effective in developing professional behaviours. Role modelling is based on learning by observation. The effects of role modelling can be increased if the role model explains the action performed (Gliatto and Stern 2013). Reflection can involve focused consideration of something observed. Teachers can assist students in reflective practice through group discussion and reflective writing including portfolios (Gliatto and

Stern 2013). These help students who may not have learnt self-assessment skills. Service learning is learning during service. Service opportunities organized by students are more effective in developing professional attitudes (Gliatto and Stern 2013).

6.8 Longitudinal Courses for Soft Skills

Longitudinal courses are better for learning soft skills than isolated courses. Ravindran et al. (1997) described teaching of ethics in an Indian medical college to undergraduate students. Didactic lectures and seminars were held weekly in the fifth semester, and case discussions involving ethical issues were held in the seventh semester. During internship, monthly sessions on cases with ethical issues covering a particular topic on clinical ethics were held.

Soft skills of communication and professionalism are part of 'professional development including ethics' course described in Medical Council of India's Regulations on Graduate Medical Education—Proposed (2012). This course has been allotted 35 h in Phase I, 35 h in Phase II, 25 h in Phase III Part 1 and 43 h in Phase III Part 2.

Altitude and Communication (AT-COM) Competencies course for the Indian Medical Graduate (Medical Council of India 2015) includes soft skills of communication, teamwork skills and bioethics. This course is spread throughout professional years of MBBS. There are five learning modules for professional year 1, eight learning modules for professional year 2, five learning modules for professional year 3 and nine learning modules for professional year 4.

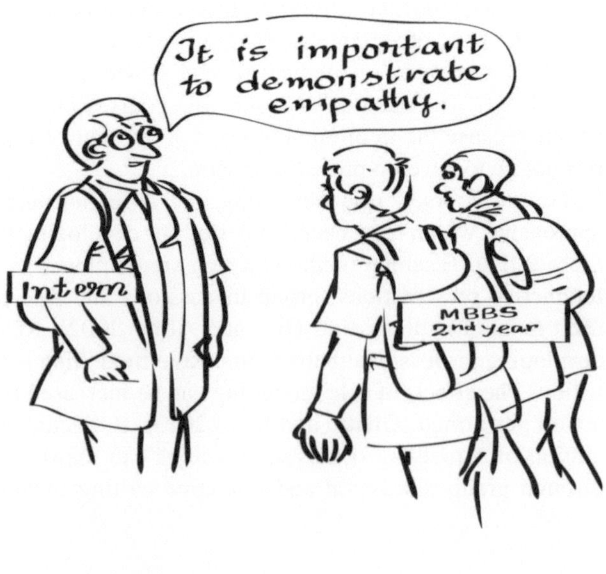
It is important to demonstrate empathy.
Intern
MBBS 2nd year

Fig. 6.2 Valuing soft skills

Conclusions

Communication skills, teamwork skills, leadership and professionalism are essential soft skills for effective functioning of medical doctors. Methods are available for developing these soft skills in medical students during undergraduate medical education. Longitudinal courses for developing soft skills are to be preferred. These courses should be integrated in undergraduate medical curriculum for optimum benefit.

References

Anon (2001) Essential elements of communication in medical encounters: the Kalamazoo consensus statement. Acad Med 76(4):390–393 Available from https://www.researchgate.net/publication/264544600_Essential_elements_of_communication_in_medical_encounters_The_Kalamazoo_Consensus_Statement. Accessed 12 Jan 2018

Anon (2002) Medical professionalism in the new millennium: a physician charter. Ann Intern Med 136(Feb):243–246. https://doi.org/10.7326/0003-4819-136-3-200202050-00012

Ber R, Alroy G (2002) Teaching professionalism with the aid of trigger films. Med Teach 24(5):528–531. https://doi.org/10.1080/0142159021000012568

Concise Oxford English Dictionary (2004) Soanes C, Stevenson A (Eds.), 11th edn. Oxford University Press Inc., New York

Core Committee, Institute for International Medical Education (2002) Global minimum essential requirements in medical education. Med Teach 24(2):130–135. PMID: 12098431. https://doi.org/10.1080/01421590220120731

Frank JR, Snell L, Sherbino J (eds) (2015) CanMEDS 2015 physician competency framework. Royal College of Physicians and Surgeons of Canada, Ottawa Available from www.royalcollege.ca/rcsite/documents/canmeds/canmeds-full-framework-e.pdf. Accessed 8 Jan 2018

Frenk J, Chen L, Bhutta ZA, Cohen J, Crisp N, Evans T et al (2010) Health professionals for a new century: transforming education to strengthen health systems in an interdependent world. Lancet 376:1923–1958. PMID: 21112623. https://doi.org/10.1016/S0140-6736(10)61854-5

General Medical Council (2015) Outcomes for graduates (Tomorrow's Doctors), July 2015. Available from https://www.gmc-uk.org/Outcomes_for_graduates_Jul_15_1216.pdf_61408029.pdf. Accessed 8 Jan 2018

Gliatto PM, Stern DT (2013) Professionalism. In: Dent JA, Harden RM (eds) A practical guide for medical teachers, 4th edn. Churchill Livingstone Elsevier, London, pp 262–269

Hamilton SS, Yuan BJ, Lachman N, Hellyer NJ, Krause DA, Hollman JH et al (2008) Interprofessional education in gross anatomy: experience with first-year medical and physical therapy students at Mayo Clinic. Anat Sci Educ 1:258–263. PMID: 19109855. https://doi.org/10.1002/ase.59

Liaison Committee on Medical Education (2016) Functions and structure of a medical school. Standards for accreditation of medical education programs leading to the M.D. degree, Mar 2016. Available from https://med.virginia.edu/ume-curriculum/wp-content/uploads/sites/216/2016/07/2017-18_Functions-and-Structure_2016-03-24.pdf. Accessed 12 Jan 2018

Losh DP, Mauksch LB, Arnold RW, Maresca TM, Storck MG, Maestas RR, Goldstein E (2005) Teaching inpatient communication skills to medical students: an innovative strategy. Acad Med 80(2):118–124 Available from http://journals.lww.com/academicmedicine/Abstract/2005/02000/Teaching_Inpatient_Communication_Skills_to_Medical.2.aspx. Accessed 12 Jan 2018

Medical Council of India (1997) Regulations on graduate medical education. Available from https://www.mciindia.org/documents/rulesAndRegulations/GME_REGULATIONS.pdf. Accessed 8 Jan 2018

Medical Council of India (2002) Indian Medical Council (Professional Conduct, Etiquette and Ethics) Regulations, 2002. Medical Council of India, New Delhi Available from https://www.mciindia.org/ActivitiWebClient/rulesnregulations/codeofMedicalEthicsRegulations2002. Accessed 8 Jan 2018

Medical Council of India (2012) Regulations on graduate medical education – proposed. Available from http://iafmonline.in/data/circular-notifications/Revised-GME-2012.pdf. Accessed 8 Jan 2018

Medical Council of India (2015) Attitude and communication (AT-COM) competencies for the Indian medical graduate. Medical Council of India, July 2015

Miles SH, Lane LW, Bickel J, Walker RM, Cassel CK (1989) Medical ethics education: coming of age. Acad Med 64:705–714 Available from http://journals.lww.com/academicmedicine/Abstract/1989/12000/Medical_ethics_education__coming_of_age.4.aspx. Accessed 12 Jan 2018

Miller GE (1990) The assessment of clinical skills/competence/performance. Acad Med 65(9):S63–S67 Available from http://winbev.pbworks.com/f/Assessment.pdf. Accessed 12 Jan 2018

Parmelee D, Hudes P, Michaelsen LK (2013) Team-based learning. In: Dent JA, Harden RM (eds) A practical guide for medical teachers, 4th edn. Churchill Livingstone Elsevier, London, pp 173–182

Ravindran GD, Kalam T, Lewin S, Pais P (1997) Teaching medical ethics in a medical college in India. Natl Med J India 10(6):288–289 Available from http://archive.nmji.in/approval/archive/Volume-10/issue-6/medical-ethics.pdf. Accessed 12 Jan 2018

Scottish Dean's Medical Education Group (2008) The Scottish Doctor: Learning outcomes for the medical undergraduate in Scotland: a foundation for competent and reflective practitioners, 3rd edn. Association for Medical Education in Europe (AMEE), Dundee Available from http://www.scottishdoctor.org/resources/scotdoc3.pdf. Accessed 8 Jan 2018

Sugand K, Abrahams P, Khurana A (2010) The anatomy of anatomy: a review for its modernization. Anat Sci Educ 3:83–93. PMID: 20205265. https://doi.org/10.1002/ase.139

Thistlethwaite JE (2013) Interprofessional education. In: Dent JA, Harden RM (eds) A practical guide for medical teachers, 4th edn. Churchill Livingstone Elsevier, London, pp 190–196

Van Staden CW, Joubert PM, Pickworth GE, Roos JL, Bergh A-M, Kruger C, Schurink WJ, Du Preez RR, Grey SV, Lindeque BG (2006) The conceptualization of "soft skills" among medical students before and after curriculum reform. S Afr Psychiatry Rev 9:33–37 Available from https://www.ajol.info/index.php/ajpsy/article/download/30205/22823. Accessed 12 Jan 2018

Vasan NS, DeFouw DO, Holland BK (2008) Modified use of team-based learning for effective delivery of medical gross anatomy and embryology. Anat Sci Educ 1:3–9. PMID: 19177372. https://doi.org/10.1002/ase.5

World Federation for Medical Education (2012) Basic Medical Education. WFME global standards for quality improvement. The 2012 revision. WFME, Copenhagen Available from http://www.um.es/documents/1935287/1936044/Revision_of_Standards_ for_Basic_Medical_Education_FINAL_260912.pdf/5866f7af-f7fc-4f9a-a7e6-eb054b7795c3. Accessed 8 Jan 2018

World Health Organization (2010) Framework for action on interprofessional educational & collaborative practice. WHO Press, World Health Organization, Geneva Available from http://apps.who.int/iris/bitstream/10665/70185/1/WHO_HRH_HPN_10.3_ eng.pdf?ua=1. Accessed 8 Jan 2018

Improving Assessments 7

I do not know of any stimulus so healthy as knowledge on the part of the student that he will receive an examination at the end of his course. It gives sharpness to his dissecting knife, heat to his Bunsen burner, a well worn appearance to his stethoscope, and a particular neatness to his bandaging.

—*William Osler, from an address to medical students at the University of Pennsylvania, 1885*

Objectives

After reading this chapter, the reader will be able to:

1. Understand the principles of designing a programme of assessment in undergraduate medical education.
2. Improve the existing assessment practices in testing knowledge and skills.

7.1 Introduction

Assessment and curriculum have been described as 'two sides of a coin'. While the curriculum lays out the plan for how learning would occur, assessment determines if it is taking place and how well. This powerful influence of assessment has led to it being labelled as 'the tail that wags the curriculum dog' and as 'the DNA of any formal education' (Tavakol and Dennick 2017). This chapter attempts to identify some of the areas in assessment in medical education that can be improved to make the discipline-based UG curriculum more effective.

Kadambari D et al., *Improving Discipline-Based Undergraduate Medical Curriculum*, https://doi.org/10.1007/978-981-13-1310-3_7

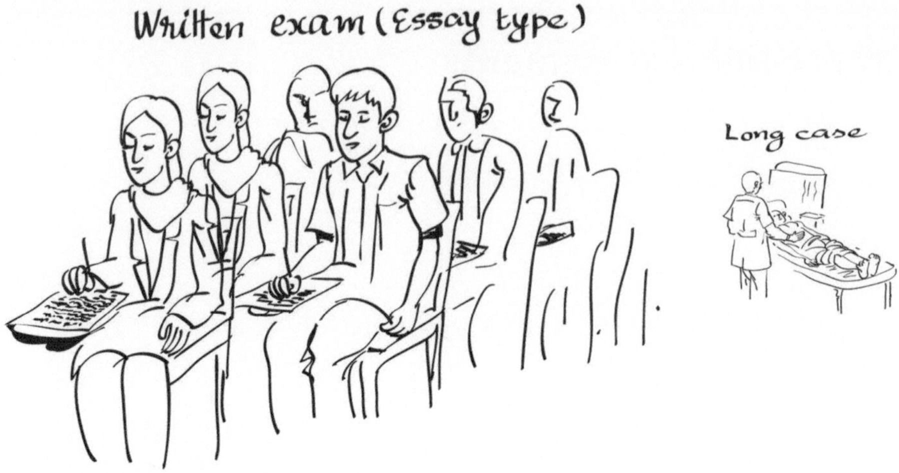

Fig. 7.1 Assessment—as it is

7.2 Purposes of Assessment

The overarching purpose of assessment is to help learning to occur, whether it is undertaken during the day-to-day interactions between student and teacher or at the end of the course. Newton (2007) identifies three levels of purposes of educational assessments. The 'judgement' level denotes the technical aim of the assessment, for example, for the purpose of making standard-referenced judgements that are usually expressed as a grade. The 'Decision' level refers to the decision/action that is taken on the basis of the judgement on assessment, for example, qualification to obtain a degree. The 'Impact' level concerns the impacts of the assessment system and is directly related to its design, for example, which all students learn the core of a subject. These levels of purposes have an implication on the design of the assessment system as we shall discuss later in the chapter. There are myriad purposes that assessments can serve. These include student monitoring, system monitoring, programme evaluation, licensing, qualification, selection, resource allocation, organizational intervention, school choice and so on (Newton 2007). From the learner's perspective, assessment data can help them choose a path in an educational programme (choose), to track their progress while identifying their strengths and weaknesses (learn) and to obtain certification or qualification (qualify). For the policy makers, assessment serves three crucial functions—to select who proceeds to the next level of learning, to monitor the functioning of various components in the system and to hold accountable those who are responsible for the components (Braun et al. 2006, p. 18).

7.3 Principles of Assessment

7.3.1 Criteria for a Good Assessment

For assessment to be judged as fulfilling its role, it must possess certain qualities. The principal criteria it must fulfil is that it should measure what it purports to measure. That is, it must have validity.

There is much debate on the conceptualization of validity in educational and psychological measurement (St-Onge et al. 2017). The generally held view is that validity refers not to the test per se but rather to the interpretation and uses or inferences drawn from the results of the assessment (Kane 2009) and that validity is determined by a process of gathering evidence to support such interpretations and uses of the measurements obtained on testing. Borsboom et al. (2004) offer a simple yet elegant concept of validity in educational testing. They distinguish between the terms 'validity' as being a property of a test and 'validation', described by Kane, as referring to an activity. In this ontological view of validity, a causal relationship exists between an attribute and the measurement scores. That is, '..... a test is valid for measuring an attribute if and only if (a) the attribute exists and (b) variations in the attribute causally produce variations in the outcomes of the measurement procedure'.

Kane (2012) proposes a framework for an argument-based approach to the validation process. This includes an interpretive argument that specifies the interpretations and uses of the test scores and a validity argument that evaluates the coherence and plausibility of the interpretive argument. The interpretive argument details the reasoning that is employed when interpreting or using scores to take decisions and must be employed each time the test scores are used. For example, interpreting the scores from checklists on an OSCE test may be quite straightforward. But when interpretation is broadened to infer clinical competence, it becomes important to decide on the tasks included (history taking, examination, communication, clinical reasoning), the scoring rules (use of checklists or global rating scales or both, including a 'critical' station) and the conditions under which the performance would occur (e.g. on simulated patients or in the workplace). Thus the broader the interpretation of measurement, the more detailed and deeper the level of evidence required (Kane 2012).

Cook et al. (2015) describe the application of Kane's validity framework in medical education. They list four inferences, scoring, generalizability, extrapolation and implications, which are included in the validity argument. Evidence needs to be collected for each of these four inferences.

Scoring inferences are derived from the translation of the observations into scores. The evidence for such inferences would be obtained from empiric evaluation of item and response option performance (item analysis data), of scoring rubrics, of rater selection, training and reliability and so on, that is, from elements in the assessment that influence scoring.

Generalizability inferences are drawn from evidence that the sample of items employed in the test is adequately representative of the 'theoretical possible items in the assessment universe' (by blueprinting and use of test specifications) and from empiric studies that would demonstrate that scores obtained on similar tests with an entirely new set of test items would generate similar scores (reproducibility).

Extrapolation inferences are derived from evidence that scores in the 'test world' are reflective of real-world performance, for example, evidence that scores reflect the level of the learner (demonstrating the expected expert-novice difference in performance).

Finally, *implication* inferences refer to the impact or consequences of assessment. Comparative studies would need to be done between groups who are and are not administering the assessment to document the impact and consequences of testing, for example, the stress levels, impact on raters or on patient care, drop-out rates and so on. Such studies, however, have limited feasibility. Other more achievable studies look at the impact of remediation, consequences of failing a test or differences in scores where they are expected to be the same, for example, between the male and female students. There are very few studies at the implications level that are in medical education literature.

There are several types of validity described. Criterion validity refers to how well the measures obtained from a test correlate with the outcome. This may refer to a comparison of summative scores in a subject discipline with the scores obtained in class tests (concurrent validity). Alternatively, it may refer to the extrapolation of the scores on a test to future performance in the domain of interest (predictive validity), e.g. evidence to show that skill performance in a simulation-based test can be extrapolated to later performance at the bedside which is obtained if the test contains samples of tasks that are expected of the graduate to be performed at the bedside.

The content of the target domain sampled by the assessment must be representative of the domain (content validity) to make appropriate interpretations. Inferences drawn from such assessments regarding the skill level in the target domain would be considered legitimate if the sample is adequately representative and wide enough to control for sampling error. Such content-based evidence alone, although indicative of relevance and representativeness, may not be sufficient for validation.

Most testing go beyond just observable performances or predictions of criteria. The test scores attempt to establish and estimate theoretical constructs or traits (e.g. clinical competence, communication skills, knowledge) that are the ultimate targets of measurement (Braun et al. 2006). Such interpretations of test scores (construct validity) involve theoretical models and claims of latent variables requiring more complex forms of evidence to be gathered.

7.3.1.1 Gathering Evidence of Validity

The *Standards for Educational and Psychological Testing* published by the American Educational Research Association (commonly referred to as the Standards) describes five sources of evidence on validity of assessments. These include evidence obtained from the content of the assessments and from the response processes and evidence based on internal structure, on the relationship to other variables and from the consequences of testing (Downing 2003; Tavakol and Dennick 2017).

Evidence from assessment content—this evidence would be gathered by a panel of subject-matter experts who would look for the representativeness of the sample content that is included in the assessment (blueprinting), the quality of the test items and the expertise of the question setter and the alignment of the test items with curricular objectives.

Evidence from response processes—this concerns evidence that all possible errors that could arise during the testing process have been eliminated or minimized. Validation evidence would include documentation of measures taken to ensure that there is adequate construct representation (blueprinting) and avoidance of construct irrelevance variance, quality control of scoring and score interpretations (use of scoring rubrics, model answers) and the accuracy of pass/fail decision rules (Downing 2003).

Evidence based on internal structure—this form of evidence includes psychometric or statistical evaluation of the test items, that is, evidence of the association between the test items and the assessment results with the construct being measured (Tavakol and Dennick 2017). Examples include item analysis data such as item discrimination and difficulty and inter-item correlation, calculation of standard error of measurement (SEM), generalizability (measure of reliability of the test scores) and differential item functioning (measurement of bias in scoring) (Downing 2003).

Evidence from the relationship to other variables—this includes correlation of test scores from two different assessments that measure the same construct, for example, a positive correlation is usually expected between scores on a summative written assessment score in anatomy with scores obtained during in-course anatomy tests (convergence) and a negative correlation between the same and scores on an OSCE test which measures a different construct (divergence).

Evidence based on consequence of tests—tests and test scores can have consequences, both positive and negative, intended or unintended. Evidence of a positive consequence may include enhanced learning among test takers, while an unintended negative consequence would occur due to a false-negative result when a deserving student fails in a high-stakes examination.

Two main threats to test validity are identified—construct underrepresentation and construct irrelevance variance. If, for example, in an assessment of clinical competence, communication skills are tested with a history-taking station in an OSCE and a few MCQs on breaking bad news, this would constitute construct underrepresentation. What would be more representative of the construct is a set of OSCE stations that assess communication in different contexts (emergency, elective), with different types of patients (co-operative, depressed, angry) and different scenarios (breaking bad news, consent for major surgery).

If performance on a computer-based test is hampered for some students who are not familiar with the use of computers, this would introduce a systematic error (bias) that would adversely affect the score of these students. Consider another situation where the examiner is particularly strict in scoring (hawk) or particularly lenient (dove), where the mean of students' scores could veer in one direction or another. In both of these examples, there is a variation in scores that is brought about by factors outside of the construct under measurement. This is referred to as construct-irrelevance variance. It could also arise due to poor testing conditions (e.g. using confusing abbreviations in the questions in a written test, not ensuring that students who have completed an OSCE test do not interact with students waiting to take the test).

Fairness is also an integral part of validity. When some among a group of students have prior knowledge of the content of the test, the scores do not truly reflect differences in performance, and their validity is undermined.

7.3.1.2 Reliability

Reliability is the consistency or reproducibility of measurements. To understand reliability it is necessary to be aware of the true score theory (Trochim 2007). According to this theory, the observed score is the true score plus error both random and systematic. The error is the source of variability from the true score. Random errors could cause variability in the measures in a random manner, for example, the effect of 'a bad day' on the performance of a student. Random errors, also termed 'noise', can inflate or deflate individual scores and add variability to the data but have little effect on the average performance of the group, as random error would be distributed normally. Systematic error on the other hand affects the entire group in the same direction, for example, when a group of students taking a test are seated in a room where the ambient noise level is high, it would affect the performance of all the test takers, and scores for the entire group could be lowered. This kind of error that affects scores of the entire group systematically in either a positive or negative direction is also termed 'bias' in measurement.

Reliability is a characteristic of a measure taken across individuals and, according to classical test theory, is estimated as the ratio of the variance of the true score (T) to the variance of the observed score (X) (where variance is calculated as the sum of the squared deviations of the scores from the mean divided by the number of scores).

That is, var.(T)/var.(X).

The above formula can be rewritten as

var.(T)/var.(T) + var.(e) where 'e' is the error.

Thus, when there is no error, $e = 0$, and the estimate of reliability is 1 (perfect reliability), and $T = X$, that is, observed score = true score. When there is no true score, only error, reliability is estimated as 0 (no reliability). A reliability coefficient of 0.8 is generally considered the minimal acceptable value (van der Vleuten and Schuwirth 2005).

But true score (T) is not a measurable entity. Hence, reliability cannot be computed. Only an estimate of reliability can be arrived at, and this is calculated as a correlation between two observations of the same measure (Trochim 2007). So, reliability like validity is related to the scores or measure and to the result or outcome of the measure, rather than the measure itself (Downing 2004).

There are four classes of reliability estimates. These include inter-rater or inter-observer reliability, test-retest reliability, parallel forms reliability and internal consistency reliability.

Inter-rater variability (variation in scores by two or more raters) can be a source of human error in reliability of measures. Examiner fatigue, distraction or misinterpretation can be causes. This can be estimated by measuring the correlation between the scores provided by the raters. For example, if we wanted to establish the inter-rater reliability on video-based performance-based assessments, we would first have a few sample videos scored by a set of raters and correlate the scores from each rater. If the correlation is high, then each rater on the team could independently rate each of the test videos, and the scores would be reliable. Inter-rater reliability can be improved by training of raters in the use of the assessment instrument.

Test-retest reliability (variability of scores arising when a test is readministered) is estimated as the level of correlation between scores obtained when the same test is administered to the same/similar sample of test takers at two points in time. Crucial to this is the time gap between the two measures, higher correlation being more likely when the gap is small and lower level of correlation when the time gap is longer. For example, if we want to estimate the test-retest reliability of video-based assessments of performance, the same rater would look at the video at two different points in time and scores correlated.

Parallel forms reliability requires the construction of parallel test forms, that is, two sets of questions that address the same construct. These are randomly administered to a set of test takers. Correlation between the two forms is an estimate of reliability. Of course, this would mean generating a lot of items that address the same construct. This form of reliability estimation is important when two tests have to be administered at two points in time, for example, when administering a supplementary test for students who have missed the regular class test.

Internal consistency reliability refers to how well items that address the same construct in a single measurement yield similar results. The correlation between scores that address the same construct (average inter-item correlation) and between items addressing the same construct and the total score on the test (average item-total correlation) is some way of estimating internal consistency reliability. Split-half reliability is similar to parallel arms reliability where items that address the same construct are divided randomly into two sets. Using pre- and post-tests can be a potential threat to the internal validity. That is, the pretest can have a teaching effect and causes the student to focus attention on the content addressed by the test items in the pretest. In such a situation, one set of items could be used for the pretest and the other for post-test. Alternatively, the two sets could be randomly assigned to the test takers in the pretest and switched in the post-test setting.

Cronbach's alpha—this is a specific measure to estimate reliability of a measure. It can be thought of as analogous to the average of all possible split-half correlations (Trochim 2007). When there are a lot of items, Cronbach's alpha is the most frequently used estimate of internal consistency.

Variability in performance across tasks is a constant observation in test takers in several subject disciplines including medical competence. In the presence of such variability across tasks, scores from tests that contain smaller samples would be unreliable measures of competence. The efficiency of the testing method in terms of time taken for a single item also influences sample size. For example, MCQ tests that take less time to solve per item can include a large sample compared to a simulation-based test that takes more time per item and therefore requires more testing time to produce reliable scores (van der Vleuten 1996). Standardization of raters and patients can minimize variability due to these factors that can threaten reliability. Using scoring rubrics for written assessments, structuring oral assessments and using multiple raters for different stations in an OSCE are some measures to reduce variability and improve reliability.

7.3.1.3 Educational Impact

Assessment drives learning. It is but natural that students aim to pass examinations and with good scores, and this provides an opportunity for test developers to reinforce desirable learning behaviour among learners (van der Vleuten 1996). It must, however, guard against the danger of the student learning to the test.

Assessment whether for or of learning influences learning. This effect is seen before (pretest), during (pure test or testing effect) and after the test (post-test) (Pugh and Regehr 2016). Before the test, whether formative or summative, the anticipation of the impending test serves as an external motivator for learning. The format of the test (example whether select or supply response) strongly influences the approach to learning, namely, rote memorization or deeper learning. Summative assessments with the higher stakes involved promoting more memorization as the aim is to pass the test (Cilliers et al. 2012). Regular, spaced out rather than only end-of-course testing has been shown to positively influence study time. Although there may be no significant influence in test scores in the short term, effects of regular testing on long-term retention have not been studied (Kerdijk et al. 2015).

Testing effect refers to the influence of the test itself beyond the impending pressure of the test. This is partly explained by the retrieval hypothesis, that is, the practice of retrieving information when undertaking the test helps the brain to develop a system to codify information in the memory (Pugh and Regehr 2016), in better retention of facts (Kroman et al. 2010) and ultimately better understanding of learnt material (Baghdady et al. 2014). Repeated testing of the same material (Karpicke and Roediger 2008) and employing construct-response questions (Kang et al. 2007) have been shown to enhance learning.

Following the test (post-test), feedback that highlights strengths and weakness has been shown to have a positive effect on learning. The feedback is made more meaningful when it is based on scores that have acceptable reliability and on tests that have sampled all areas of the domain sufficiently to identify areas that need improvement (Pugh and Regehr 2016). The credibility of the feedback determines its acceptability to the receiver as does its focus on the task rather than on the person.

Other criteria of good assessments include acceptability and costs/resources, fairness, transparency, meaningfulness and so on. Assessments must be acceptable to both examiners and test takers. There could be a reluctance to accept newer assessment methods in an educational system where tradition holds sway, as in medical education, even when there is evidence to support its use (van der Vleuten

1996). This may be particularly applicable in the summative setting with its high stakes where assessments need to be defensible. Cost and other resources required for an assessment also have a significant influence on its implementability. However valid or reliable the scores from an assessment, if it is resource intensive for the individual institute, it will not be sustainable.

van der Vleuten (1996) describes the concept of utility of an assessment, which he derives as the multiplicative product of these five characteristics, namely, the classical criteria of validity, reliability and education effects along with the criteria of acceptability and cost/feasibility. The utility index so derived is more of a conceptual model than an actual mathematical algorithm. Each of these criteria has a different weightage that would depend on the context and purpose of the assessment. For instance, a high-stakes summative exam would require a high level of reliability compared to a low-stakes class assessment. Also, the use of a multiplicative formula means that if any of the criteria is absent (value = 0), the assessment has zero utility.

7.4 The Formative Purpose of Assessment

The use of assessment data to identify learner weaknesses and strengths and to modify teaching strategies fits the description of its formative purpose. Thus, the judgement from an assessment is being used for a certain purpose, that is, supporting learning in its context, for instance, in the classroom or during a bedside case discussion. Feedback to the learner that clarifies her goals, where she stands with respect to those goals and on strategies to get there is at the core of formative assessment (Black and Wiliam 2009). The sources of this feedback include the teacher, peers and the learner herself. In work-based contexts such as in medical education, feedback may be obtained from other sources as well (Yorke 2005).

7.4.1 Importance of Formative Assessment

FA can be viewed as a strategy by the teacher to bridge the gap between educational goals and the learner with a view to reducing the error component of trial and error in learning (Sadler 1998). It is also seen as a move to redirect the attention of assessment from high-stakes external testing on scores and grades to low-stakes assessment that is focused on raising the standards of education (Black and William 2010).

7.4.2 How, When and Where Do We Do It?

Black and Wiliam (2009) identify the following as five key strategies that conceptualize the formative purpose of assessments:

1. Clarifying and sharing learning intentions and criteria for success.
2. Engineering effective classroom discussions and other learning tasks that elicit evidence of student understanding.

3. Providing feedback that moves learners forward.
4. Activating students as instructional resources for one another.
5. Activating students as the owners of their own learning.

A key issue in the practice of formative assessment is the nature of the dialogue between the teacher and learner. In a typical dialogue between the teacher and student in a classroom, the teacher asks a question (initiation) and the learner provides an answer (response) which the teacher evaluates and reacts to (evaluation), thus setting up an interaction that has been termed I-R-E. It is a common practice among teachers that when they pose a question to a class, the question requires the learner to fill in a missing word or phrase, by which the teacher is steering the learner towards the expected answer. In the formative mode, however, the teacher's initial task aims to encourage more thought in the learner whose response creates a more unpredictable reaction in the teacher. In other words, the teacher is trying to understand the thinking process in the learner and her reaction, rather than giving a predictable direction to the learner which will be contingent on the learner's response. This understanding of the learner's cognitive processes is necessary for providing effective formative feedback. So, in a classroom interaction, the teacher has two tasks to perform in a very short time—diagnostic, which is to understand the thinking process in the learner, and prognostic, which is to provide the optimum response.

A relevant action to be performed by the learner in a classroom setting is self-assessment for which she should be aware of the goals or standards that are to be reached. Black and Wiliam (2009) evoke Winne and Hadwin's self-regulated learning (SRL) model to explain a learner's response to a classroom task. In this model the learner begins by identifying the task, a step that is strongly influenced by her domain knowledge. Next, she plans a response and then enacts a strategy which she adapts as the task proceeds. Other conditions could influence this response including her prior experiences, motivation, beliefs and task conditions including resources, time and local context.

Although such 'mutually hermeneutic exchanges' between teacher and learner (Yorke 2005) form the core activity in formative assessment, the learning taking place in the classroom is essentially under the teacher's control. She has the responsibility of creating the situations that would provide maximum opportunities for learners to learn and/or develop learning autonomy. It is also her task to keep the learners on the right track to achieving the learning aims of the discipline.

The third player in the practice of formative assessment is the group of peers. The concept of assessment and feedback from peers has grown in higher education contexts. van der Pol et al. (2008) define it 'as a method in which students engage in reflective criticism of the products of other students and provide them with feedback, using previously defined criteria'. Peer assessment has a positive influence on the assessor's own self-assessment skills, but from the perspective of the receiver, the credibility (senior versus a peer at the same level of learning) and the feedback providing ability including domain knowledge of the giver are major factors that influence its acceptance. Some of these issues can be tackled with training students and incorporating peer assessment as an essential component in the overall assessment practices.

7.4.3 The Place of Feedback

Feedback occupies a central position in formative assessment practice. Ramaprasad (1983) has defined it as follows:

> Feedback is information about the gap between the actual level and the reference level of a system parameter which is used to alter the gap in some way.

Assessment feedback encompasses all feedback exchanges that are included in the design of assessments including those that occur within and outside the context of the assessments, whether actively or passively sought or received and from various sources (Evans 2013). Assessment feedback can motivate (influence beliefs), provide reinforcement (reward or punish behaviours) or be informational (taking learning in a certain direction) (Nelson and Schunn 2009).

Seen from a socio-constructive view, feedback is facilitative, that is, through comments and suggestions, the learner revises her work and, through dialogue, develops new understandings (Archer 2010). The teacher's feedback comprises of three core processes (Sadler 1998). First, the teacher provides the stimulus for the student to produce the result of her learning (for instance, assigning a written task). Second, the teacher assesses this against a reference framework, a step that identifies the strengths and weaknesses. As the third step, the teacher provides an explicit judgement in the form of a grade, a mark or a statement on the quality of the work that justifies the judgement along with suggestions to improve. Such feedback could include providing (non-evaluative) descriptions of the features of the work, evaluative comments that are linked to criteria and which indicate those features of the work that add to or detract from high quality and suggestions for alternative ways that the work could have been done that would have led to improvement in order to be able to provide such feedback the teacher draws on her resources that include her expertise in the subject domain and its assessment, her attitudes towards teaching, her skill at constructing the assessment tasks, her knowledge of the criteria and standards that are appropriate for the tasks, her expertise at forming a judgement of the student's work and her ability to provide feedback. The teacher's knowledge of a student's past experiences and achievement levels helps her to tailor the feedback to a particular student.

In a more complex scenario, the learning and feedback can be bidirectional between teacher and learner that can be mutually beneficial—a co-constructivist view. Feedback as it corrects subscribes to a cognitivist view and is termed directive. Feedback in assessment must incorporate both elements.

Hattie and Timperley (2007) identify four types of feedback—focusing on clarifying and reinforcing aspects of the learning task (task feedback); on what the learner does to proceed with the learning task (process feedback); on the metacognitive aspects of learning, that is, monitoring and evaluating strategies employed by the learner (self-regulation feedback); or on how well the learner performs the task (self-feedback). Each of these has a variable impact on the learning gain with process and task feedback having a greater effect than self-feedback.

Evans (2013) identifies the following principles of effective feedback:

1. Feedback is ongoing and an integral part of assessment—feedback is an integral part of the assessment and not seen in isolation.
2. Assessment feedback guidance is explicit—guidance is explicit on the assessment and on expectations in terms of quality.
3. Greater emphasis is placed on feedforward compared to feedback activities—timely feedback which also guides on future tasks.
4. Students are engaged in and with the process—students make their own improvement plans and are empowered to 'think for themselves'.
5. The technicalities of feedback are attended to in order to support learning—feedback focuses on the performance of the task, identifies strategies for improvement and encourages interaction and dialogue.
6. Training in assessment feedback/forwards is an integral part of assessment design—training of teachers, learners (to self-assess) and peers (in peer assessment and peer feedback).

Merely providing feedback does not mean that the learner will use it (Sadler 1989). A feedback gap arises when students are unable to capitalize on feedback even when it is good. Individual variations in perceptions of feedback between the learner and teacher, in the ability to give and receive feedback and impact of the context and relationship between the feedback provider and recipient, are some contributors to the gap. Feedback even when task-based involves emotional and motivational reactions which must be kept in mind when attempting to take learning forward with feedback (Stobart 2012).

7.5 Improving Assessments

7.5.1 Improving Test Design

If we agree that the principle aim of assessment in education is to enhance learning, then we must shift the focus away from assessment of learning to assessment for learning. If assessment is for learning, the design of the assessment must reflect this. In most higher education contexts, traditional assessments have a measurement orientation, that is, they are focused on 'reliable performance of individuals on decontextualised, standardised tasks that are deemed to be valid indicators of the domain being assessed' and are aimed at establishing individual differences (MacLellan 2001). The standards-based model, on the other hand, employs authentic tasks to establish the level of knowledge that is based on deep understanding of the domain. Mislevy et al. (2003) proposes an evidentiary model of test design (evidence-centred design, ECD) that begins with determining the claims that assessment users would like to make (i.e. the purpose or use of the assessment judgements) and the evidence required to establish those claims. Then the exercises to elicit desired learner responses can be developed, that is, the test items, followed by the development of scoring rubrics that would translate the responses into evidence and the measurement models that summarize the evidence. Advances in technology have increased the means of gathering evidence, for instance, with the use of simulations and computer-based testing.

Judgements made on performance in assessments range from summative decisions on the quality or level of competence in the domain and characterized by appraisal to descriptive judgements reflecting the nature of the competence by a process of analysis (Newton 2007). The summative end of this continuum is essentially quantitative judgements that are made with respect to previous performance by self (self-referenced) or with respect to performance of the group (norm-referenced). The descriptive end of the continuum is judgements that are qualitative inferences of educational attainment. Between the two extremes of the continuum are standard-referenced judgments and criterion-referenced judgements. Judgements based on educational standards are usually expressed in quantitative terms, for example, a score of 80% would mean that the student has attained 80% of the set performance standards. These judgements are aided by the setting of explicit criteria of performance. Thus, criteria could be considered descriptors of standards. Judgements based on criteria would then be explicit statements of the attainment of the student, that is, what she can and cannot do, for example, palpates the abdomen correctly but makes errors during percussion or the answer on a written test contains a comprehensive treatment plan for a given patient but does not address rehabilitative measures.

When designing an assessment, the first step would be to describe what is valued in the domain of interest, that is, the knowledge and performance outcomes, the task features and knowledge-task relationships and so on.

This is followed by organizing this information about the domain according to what claims are to be made about the students and the proficiency level (e.g. selecting tasks at various difficulty levels), the evidence that is to be gathered to support the claim (e.g. scoring rubrics) and the tasks that will be employed to gather this evidence (viz. written or performance tasks).

The selected tasks must match the domain of interest, for example, using an OSCE station to test communication skills or using a written test of MCQs to test factual knowledge.

Miller (1990) described a conceptual model for assessment of clinical competence (Fig. 7.2).

The broad domain of knowledge is addressed at two levels at the base of the pyramid—the 'knows' and 'knows how' levels. Written tests employing various tools such as essay items, MCQs, key feature problems (Page et al. 1995) and oral examinations (viva) provide validity to measures these two levels. Performance in the contrived situation of the examination setting ('shows how') is assessed with tools such as OSCE stations, the traditional long case, while the apex of the pyramid is performance at the 'does' level that refers to actual performance in the workplace. A valid measure at this level would require evidence that is challenging to collect and would include evidence of improved health parameters in the clinician's practice. The workplace-based assessment measures occur in the workplace but suffer

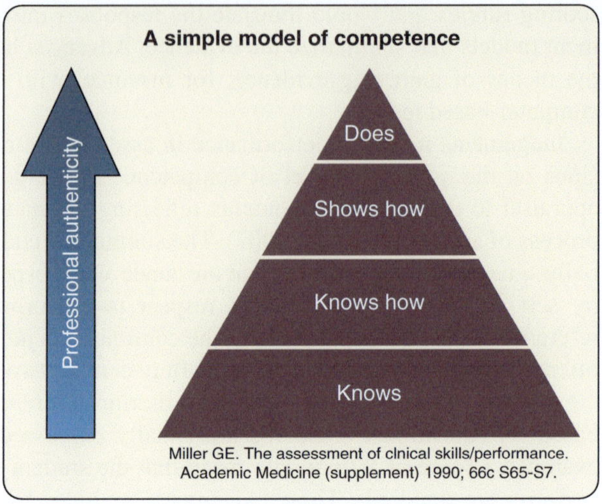

Fig. 7.2 Miller's Triangle

from reliability issues when used to make summative judgements. Although Miller's model of assessment strategies provides a guide to the selection of the tool for the assessment of the various subcomponents of clinical competence, it does not take into account the interplay between the various aspects of competence and the need for a composite measurement method (Dijkstra et al. 2010).

We will keep referring to Miller's pyramid of assessment strategies in further sections of the chapter.

7.5.2 Making Defensible Summative Judgements

7.5.2.1 Standard Setting

Assessments that make a summative judgement for qualification should be able to differentiate competent from non-competent test takers. This is achieved with the use of a 'cut score' that is arrived at by a process termed standard setting. We have already talked about norm-referenced and criterion-referenced judgements. With the use of norm-referenced standards, the passing scores are relative, that is, performance of the student is relative to the performance of the entire group. Thus, the cut score will be determined by the number of students who will pass, for example, selecting all those with scores above the 70th percentile into a medical school. Thus, the passing score would vary with each examination. Standards are not set in advance, and diagnostic feedback relative to performance will be unclear (Friedman Ben-David 2000). Norm-referenced standards are suitable to assessments for selection where a fixed number of positions are available (McKinley and Norcini 2014).

When the passing score is predetermined (e.g. at 50% for assessments of clinical skills) and remains the same for all subsequent tests, the appropriateness of the passing score is adversely affected as the difficulty level could vary with each examination, as can the items in the test. With the use of criterion-referenced standards, pass/fail rates will vary with each year as the criteria are absolute.

Compensatory standards refer to the process by which the standard is set at the level of the total score across items. So poor performance in one set of items can be compensated by better performance in others. This may not be applicable in assessments of clinical competence where more than one method is being employed and more than one construct is being assessed. For example, in an OSCE exam, a test taker may do poorly in history taking but may be able 'compensate' by doing very well in physical examination. Conjunctive standards, in contrast, require that a certain number of stations have to be competently managed in order for a test taker to be declared pass. Conjunctive standards may lead to unreliable pass/fail decisions if there is a measurement error in any of the stations.

Broadly there are two models of standard setting methods—test-centred and examinee-centred (Friedman Ben-David 2000). In test-centred models, a panel of judges (subject experts) review the test items and decide what would be the 'just acceptable' level of performance on the test. The panel of judges usually comprises about ten experts (ranging from 5 to 20 in several studies) (Hejri and Jalili 2014), who have varying levels of experience in the subject and in the testing method and are at varying levels of expertise. Through discussion and consensus, the panel decides on how many items will be passed by a 'borderline' (this must not be equated with 'average') student. The Angoff model is popular in educational settings and is employed in the Ebel and Nedelsky methods. Test-centred standard setting occurs before the test is conducted.

In the examinee-centred model, such as the borderline and borderline-regression methods, the panel of judges review the performance of the group of students on the test to determine the borderline group and the cut score. The borderline group is thus not hypothetical, and the pass-fail decision is made by the judges by selecting a point on the score scale that is matched to the purpose of the test (Friedman Ben-David 2000).

Standard setting methods are criticized for the subjectivity (judgement of experts with risk of disagreement), the challenge in defining the minimum competency student and the variability of the standard setting results when different methods are used.

7.5.2.2 Use of Scoring Rubrics

A scoring rubric is 'a scoring tool for qualitative rating of authentic or complex student work' (Jonsson and Svingby 2007). It serves as a guide for the assessor to know what is important when assessing a student's performance and can be used for both high-stakes and classroom assessments. The rubric may be holistic, where the scoring is a generic judgement of the overall quality of the assessment, or analytic, where the assessor assigns a separate score for each dimension of the assessment task. Holistic scoring rubrics are easier to use in large-scale assessments, while analytic scoring rubrics are preferred for classroom assessments where the purpose is to identify students' strengths and weaknesses. For example, an analytic rubric for assessing a short essay may look at the dimensions of content, organization, development and use of language. Specific levels of success for each element are then delineated, that is, from poorest to best. Ratings are then assigned to the various levels and a scoring system devised. A rubric can be generic or task specific.

Scoring with rubrics improves inter-rater reliability. This is seen more with the use of analytic and task-specific rubrics which also contain exemplars for the different levels (Jonsson and Svingby 2007).

7.5.3 Programmatic Approach to Assessment Design

The predominant pattern of testing in higher education settings has been the single 'summing up' assessment at the end of the course. This has several unintended consequences such as a learner's perception of the 'sting' of social judgement that accompanies a pass-fail decision (Pugh and Regehr 2016; Cilliers et al. 2012). This results in a shift of the learner's orientation towards succeeding in the test with superficial strategies such as rote memorization rather than on learning with understanding. This could also be accompanied by undesirable practices such as cheating. From the perspective of the teacher, the focus could shift to 'teaching to the test' (a not too uncommon scenario in many settings across the world!). Additionally, there is little scope for providing meaningful feedback for remediation. These issues could be addressed with a programme of assessment that runs through the entire educational course and that is predominantly aimed at improving learning.

This approach to assessment design consists of combining various assessment methods at different points in time during the training programme, each such assessment constituting a data point. Rather than using a single end-of-course assessment result to make a decision, in such a longitudinal design of assessment, the information from several such data points gathered over time is synthesized to provide information on the competence level of the learner (Dijkstra et al. 2010).

With a clearly defined goal, informed, rational decisions can be made about the assessment areas needed to be included, the methods to be employed, how the results from various sources will be combined and the balancing of the strengths and weaknesses of the programme's components. The benefits of this approach would be the combination of various instruments, the move to go beyond the assessment of 'easy-to-measure' elements such as factual knowledge, and basing high-stakes decisions on more than one source to make well-informed highly defensible decisions (Dijkstra et al. 2010). Therefore, one competency domain is assessed using different methods, and the results from one method can address more than one competency domain (Schuwirth and van der Vleuten 2011). It is noteworthy that there is no 'bad' assessment method just as there is no ideal one.

Dijkstra et al. (2010) proposes a framework for a programme of assessment that begins with identification of the purpose of the assessment. The purpose or goals of assessment are the key factor that determines the structure of the programme. Hence the guiding principle of a programmatic approach is 'fitness for purpose'. This step is followed by the 'programme in action' that comprises of collecting and valuing information and taking appropriate action. This refers to the processes of determining the content, the selection and use of the assessment format and instrument, the scoring system to be employed and the scheduling of the assessment. This phase is directed at collecting information on the learner's abilities in the form of numeric (quantitative) and/or descriptive (qualitative) data. The information so gathered is then integrated and interpreted (valuing information) to take some decision (taking action), whether pass-fail or identification of the learner's strengths and weaknesses or prioritization of learning goals.

The framework next includes supporting actions taken to maintain a high standard for the programme in action. This includes technical support measures that would contribute to enhancing the quality of the instruments, such as review of the test items before administering them and post hoc psychometric analysis for improvement and training of assessors. Legal and political support would also be required to ensure acceptability of the programme by the stakeholders.

Documentation forms the next component in the framework and is a step taken to make the assessment programme more defensible as well as for improvement. The context and applicability of the programme as also the rules and regulations that will provide stakeholders the information on how it would affect them must be clearly laid down. A third important element to be documented is the blueprint that maps the content of the domain to the programme and the instruments to be used.

The loop is closed with research and development that aids in a continuous improvement cycle. Any proposals to modify the programme based on research findings are best managed by employing the appropriate change management techniques.

The increasing need to build a defensibility to assessment decisions is also recognized in the framework. Using appropriate research findings to inform decisions, employing external reviewers and ensuring cost-effectiveness are some of the strategies listed.

The programmatic approach to assessment in medical education has been attempted in different contexts (Dannefer and Henson 2007; Lew et al. 2002; Van der Vleuten et al. 2017). van der Vleuten et al. (2017) describe their experience with a programme of assessment for learning, in which the assessments are all low-stakes ones. The programme combines several instruments such as MCQ tests, assignments, open-ended question formats, projects, etc. for the module assessments in the first 2 years of a PBL curriculum. During the clinical rotations, they employ workplace-based assessments (Norcini and Burch 2007) such as miniCEX, OSATS and MSF instruments. A longitudinal cross-modular assessment uses the progress test (Tio et al. 2016) that tests learners at all levels in the programme with the same set of 200 questions four times a year. For the 'soft skills' component of clinical competence, peer and tutor assessment with feedback is employed. The student is given access to all information about their assessments which is stored on an e-portfolio. This programme of assessment which begun with the graduate training programme with an annual intake of 50 students has been extended to the undergraduate programme taking in 340 students each year.

Another approach to design assessment for learning is with the use of entrustable professional activities (Peters et al. 2017). Initially used to design assessments of competence in postgraduate education, they have been expanded for use in undergraduate training. The underlying principle in the use of EPAs is that attainment of competence is related to opportunities for learning that are determined by the level of trust in the learner by the teacher. A learner passes through phases of learning when he/she cannot be trusted for any task through a graded increase in the trust level accompanying a gradual decrease in supervision by the tutor to reach the final level of independent practice when she can be trusted to supervise others.

7.5.4 Improving Written Assessments

Written assessments have had a place in the medical education setting for a long time and are used for assessing competence at the level of 'knows' and 'knows how' of Miller's pyramid. The pendulum has swung from the use of essays to MCQs to counter some of the problems associated with the use of essays and back to believing that there is a role for construct-response type of written test format in medical education. This section of the chapter, rather than describing individual tools used for written assessments, will attempt to discuss some of the common misconceptions, problems in the use of some frequently used test formats such as MCQs and on how to address these problems.

Written assessments can be broadly categorized as supply-/constructed-response formats (essays, short answer questions, fill in the blanks) and selected-response formats (MCQs, match the following). Another categorization is into response format and stimulus format (Schuwirth and van der Vleuten 2004), the latter referring to the stimulus provided by the content of the question for the thought process in the test taker, for example, with the use of a case scenario.

Although MCQ-based tests are now the most commonly used format of examinations, both for selection and licensing purposes in medical education, essays are still being used in many settings. Essays provide an insight into the thinking process in the student. In the context of medical education therefore, where problem-solving is the core skill to be developed, they offer a useful measure of the clarity of thought and a logical informed approach to problem-solving. But essays are notoriously time taking to score and could be associated with reduced reliability due to variations in the scoring by the same or different assessors. The validity of the measure is also affected adversely by construct-irrelevance variance introduced by the marker's fatigue arising from the large number of answers to be assessed, his disagreement with the content and the way it has been presented by the learner as well as any biases related to gender, ethnicity and so on. Additionally, within the time available for testing, essays (or for the matter any of the constructed-response formats) sample a much smaller portion of the discipline content compared to MCQs. Hence, in large-scale high-stakes assessments, MCQs could provide more reliable scores than essays.

Some misconceptions are common regarding the use of essays (Reiner et al. 2002). For instance, they always test higher-order and critical thinking skills. In truth this is determined by the content of the question than the format itself. Consider the question as follows:

Classify lymphoma. Write in detail about clinical features, diagnosis and management of Hodgkin's lymphoma.

This question does not require the student to demonstrate her reasoning or analytical ability, nor does it test whether she is able to select the optimum treatment approach for a given patient with Hodgkin's lymphoma.

Consider the question reframed as follows:

A 24-year-old lady presents with a painless swelling on one side of her neck that she noticed has been growing since 4 weeks. On examination you find that she has bilateral firm cervical lymphadenopathy. What other clinical findings will help you to arrive at a diagnosis? How will you confirm your clinical suspicion?

Although the reframed question requires the student to list out the clinical features from memory, it at least provides a context for it, which requires some analysis. If the objective being tested is the selection of an appropriate treatment regime, the scenario in the question could provide the diagnosis and require the student to formulate a treatment plan.

Let us look at another example, this time from the basic sciences.

Describe the anatomy of the femoral triangle.

Compare this to the following:

With the help of a suitable diagram, explain how intra-abdominal contents can herniate into the femoral region. What structures are at risk of damage when operating in this region?

In each of the examples given, the revised version requires the question setter to align the content of the question to the learning outcome that is intended to be tested, for example, arriving at a clinical diagnosis in a patient presenting with cervical lymphadenopathy or understanding the clinical relevance of studying the anatomy of the femoral region, both of which fall into the higher levels of application of knowledge.

The second misconception is that essay items are easy to construct. As we can see from the examples given above, questions that assess higher-order thinking skills are not easy to frame.

A third misconception is that in contrast to MCQs, essays eliminate guessing. This may not be entirely true. It brings in guessing of a different nature—bluffing.

A fourth misconception is that essays require students to prepare more thoroughly. However, it has been shown that more than the format of the test, what influences preparation by the student is what is expected of her, that is, the cognitive complexity of the task (Crooks 1988).

MCQs of the single best response type are ubiquitous. The well-known advantage of using MCQs includes the ease of administration and marking especially in large-scale assessments and the wider sampling of the domain that enhances the reliability of the scores. If constructed well, they can also be used to test knowledge at a higher level of Bloom's taxonomy. However, just as with essays, good MCQs are not easy to design and are time-consuming to create. Items that test at the level of recall of facts are easy to construct and tend to predominate in a test. With the use of computers, large-scale testing can employ computer algorithms for automated item generation (Gierl et al. 2012). Item models are created from cognitive models that are developed by content specialists. New items are developed from these item models using computer software.

Other limitations are that writing good distractors is hard work and the student may often resort to 'recognizing' the answer without actually knowing or reasoning it out (guessing) which means that the selected option by the student does not give an insight into her thinking, that is, the scorer is not able to understand the reasoning behind the choice.

Several technical flaws may arise when constructing MCQs (Case et al. 1996). These include issues related to test-wiseness such as the presence of grammatical and logical cues, the correct option being longer, use of absolute terms like 'always' and 'never' in the options and issues of irrelevant difficulty such as the use of an unnecessarily complicated stem or options that are vague and poorly written.

The quality of MCQs can be improved with the following measures (Case et al. 1996):

1. Employing the 'cover the options' rule, that is, the clarity of the task in the stem is such that the student should be able to answer the item without looking at the options.
2. Keeping the options short with a longer stem.
3. Avoiding superfluous information both in the stem and the options.
4. Avoiding the use of overly complex items.
5. Ensuring that options are grammatically consistent and logically compatible with the stem, that they are of the same relative length as the key and that they are plausible and listed in a logical or alphabetical order.
6. Avoiding vague terms ('usually' or 'commonly') and absolute terms ('always', 'never') in the options.
7. Avoiding negatives in the stem as far as possible.

When constructing single best-answer type of MCQs in the basic sciences, a patient vignette can be used to assess application of basic science knowledge to clinical medicine. For example, when the question is about the area of the brain that is supplied by a certain artery, a clinical vignette that describes the consequences of occlusion of the artery can be used. Alternatively, a lab vignette that gives the results of a lab test could require the student to interpret the results. Constructing such items would call for dialogues between teachers from basic science and clinical disciplines.

For items in clinical sciences that attempt to test at a higher level of knowledge than recall of facts, the student may be required to make a choice from a list of possible diagnoses, investigations, treatment options, mechanisms of disease and so on. Although the use of scenarios has no significant effect on the discrimination and difficulty level compared to non-vignette questions, they require the student to go beyond memorization of a large body of facts by providing information that requires analysis and application (Case et al. 1996).

Other formats of written test that could be used to test at a higher level of knowledge include the extended matching type of MCQs (Case and Swanson 2001), key feature problems (to test clinical decision-making skills) (Page et al. 1995; Page 1999) and script concordance test questions (Charlin et al. 1998; Lubarsky et al. 2013). Detailed descriptions of these formats are available in the quoted references, and the reader is encouraged to refer to them for the design and use of these formats.

When trying to decide whether an essay item is to be used rather than an MCQ, taking into consideration the directive verb employed in the objective that is being assessed helps (Reiner et al. 2002). For example, with verbs such as 'explain', 'defend', 'analyse', 'evaluate' and 'compose' in an objective, the student would be required to construct her response. In contrast, with verbs such as 'identify', 'match', 'classify', 'recognize' and so on, the student could select the answer from a list of options.

The use of essays in high-stakes summative assessments may be associated with problems of reliability and validity (Hift 2014). But in the assessment-for-learning setting, essays and other form of written assessments such as assignments and projects provide the teacher an insight into the thinking process in the student. This enables her to provide high-quality feedback to help the student identify her strengths and weaknesses and devise strategies to improve. Where reliability is crucial, such as end-of-module assessments, high-quality select response types of questions that test knowledge beyond recall and which have a larger sampling of the content would be more appropriate.

An attempt at bringing in integration of course content needs to be complemented with integrative 'cross-course' assessments (Swanson and Case 1997). That is, assessments should test the student's ability to integrate her knowledge in the different disciplines. A few such items could be included in the summative examination and the scores obtained on them divided among the subjects addressed.

7.5.5 Improving Performance-Based Assessments

Clinical and procedural skills assessment falls into the 'shows how' (in the setting of an examination) and 'does' (at the workplace) levels of Miller's pyramid.

Traditionally, clinical skills have been assessed with a long case and short case format of testing which is still followed in many clinical training settings. The long case examination has come under criticism for several reasons (Wass et al. 2001).

The main issue with the use of the long case is the poor reliability or reproducibility of the scores. That is, performance on one case does not predict performance on another. Studies have demonstrated reproducibility coefficients in tests employing two long cases to be as low as 0.39, which means that only 39% of the score was due to variability in student performance and 61% was due to 'noise' (measurement errors) (Norcini 2002). The most important reason for the low reproducibility is the problem of case specificity. It is known that physicians perform differently on different patient problems and that there are several factors that account for this. In other words, problem-solving is not a generic skill. What is required therefore is to assess the learner over a range of patient problems to generalize to typical performance. A second reason is examiner variability. When experts assess learner performance, their scoring is influenced by their own level of knowledge, their beliefs and perceptions of what constitutes the right approach to a given problem as well as personal biases. This is compounded by variability in the behaviour of the patients with different test takers.

Very often the patient encounter in a long case examination is not observed, which can be a threat to the validity of scores.

Despite these criticisms, it is acknowledged that the long case is a tool that captures an authentic clinical encounter between the learner and a patient which lends the measure of its validity. All aspects of clinical competence, including clinical skills such as history taking, physical examination and diagnostic reasoning, communication skills and professionalism can be assessed with the long case encounter. Observation of the encounter enhances the validity of the measure, for example, with the use of the Objective Structured Clinical Examination Record (OSLER) (Gleeson 1997). To increase its reliability, several long cases have to be employed which would lead to an unrealistic increase in test time.

The issues of low reliability associated with the long case are addressed by the Objective Structured Clinical Examinations (OSCEs) (Harden and Gleeson 1979). A typical summative OSCE examination will consist of 10–20 stations that sample across a wide range of clinical competencies including procedural skills (e.g. peripheral venous cannulation). In many settings, standardized patients are used particularly for scoring performance in a communication skills station. Their use in stations testing other aspects of clinical competence such as history taking and physical examination is limited by the complexity of the problems that they need to portray (Norcini 2002). Rigorous training of the SPs is required to improve the metrics of scores on stations employing them. Generally, 10–20% of scoring is contributed by SP ratings (Pell et al. 2010). Another perceived advantage of the OSCE is the 'objectivity' in contrast to the subjective or holistic scoring used for a long case assessment. Schuwirth and van der Vleuten (2011) reiterate the importance of 'subjective' human judgement in the assessment of clinical competence. The dichotomous scoring with the use of checklists does not capture the quality of performance by the student and is better combined with a global rating scale.

But OSCEs are expensive and resource (space, raters, SPs) intensive, especially in the high-stakes summative setting. Other criticisms levelled at the OSCE are the risk of atomization of competencies which could result in sacrificing validity for reliability and objectivity.

As with all assessments, quality lies with the way it is used. Standard setting to define cut scores is an important step in the planning of an OSCE summative exam. Examinee-centred methods such as the borderline-regression method (McKinley and Norcini 2014) are preferred to test-centred methods such as the Angoff technique.

The internal consistency of the OSCE test, measured as Cronbach's alpha, can be reduced with the use of too few stations or poorly designed items or if items in a given set measure different constructs or if assessors are not measuring to a common standard (Pell et al. 2010). Some other quality metrics include measuring the coefficient of determination R^2, which is a measure of the correlation of the checklist score with the global rating scoring in each station, with the expectation that higher overall global rating should generally correspond with higher checklist scores. Failure rates on a station, intergroup variance including assessor effects ('hawks' or 'doves'), site (context) effects and the effect of standardized patient scorings are some of the other measures of quality of OSCE that are useful for quality improvement.

Thus, in the assessment of clinical competence, no single method or instrument is 'perfect'. Instead, a longitudinal programme of assessment employing methods that combine the benefits while reducing the shortcomings of each other is recommended. The purpose of the assessment would determine the choice of instrument. For continuous in-training assessments, the OSLER is a valid instrument that also provides opportunity for feedback. For formative purposes, workplace-based tools such as the miniCEX, Direct Observation of Procedural Skills and case-based discussions provide valid measures of skills that can form the basis for feedback and remediation. Although WPBA tools provide valid information regarding the performance of the trainees in various aspects of their learning, implementation faces some important challenges. Difficulty in finding assessors, variability in the perceived usefulness of the different tools from the perspective of students, inconsistency with which immediate feedback is provided are some of the issues that have been noted (Quantrill and Tun 2012). OSCEs are useful at all stages of training. During the early phases, 'teaching OSCEs' accompanied by remedial feedback are useful for learning component clinical skills. As the learner progresses, checklists can be replaced with global rating scales that provide an overall measure of competence.

7.6 Quality Assurance of the Assessment Programme

The importance of building an accountable programme of assessment cannot be overemphasized. The medical education community has the responsibility of ensuring that the students graduating from a medical school are competent doctors. Passing underperformers happens quite frequently in medical education (Dudek et al. 2005). This is undesirable, as underperformers could be incompetent doctors with a detriment to society.

The quality of the assessment programme can be improved by training assessors, focusing the purpose of assessments on improving learning, standardizing high-stakes tests with the use of standard setting and post hoc item analysis and continuous evaluation of the assessment programme with post-examination analysis of assessment data.

We have considered the need for and some common methods of standard setting in an earlier section of the chapter. The statistical testing involved in item analysis and assessment of examination data are beyond the scope of this chapter, and the reader is referred to detailed guides on the topics for further reading (Pell et al. 2010; Tavakol and Dennick 2011; Tavakol and Dennick 2012).

7.7 Training of Assessors

Human judgement has a key role to play in assessment of competence. However, rater-based assessments are fallible and face difficulties including inaccuracy in observation, rating biases (e.g., halo error), inconsistency in rating, failure to identify deficiencies and difficulty discriminating between dimensions (Tavares and Eva 2013). These problems have highlighted the need for training assessors to increase their awareness of such biases (Schleicher et al. 2017).

Although it is believed that training may address some of the common issues that threaten validity and reliability of measurements (Green and Holmboe 2010), studies have shown varying results of training. The training process must aim at improving the use of the various measurement tools available. For example, a programme to train assessors in OSCEs could comprise a course during which they are made aware of the principles and underlying philosophy of OSCEs, provided practice opportunities in scoring (for instance, on videos of performances) or on role playing as assesses and in standard setting methods to determine cut scores (Pell et al. 2008). Giving and receiving quality feedback are other areas that training programs can have an impact on the assessment-for-learning programme.

However, the value of professional judgement that is brought in especially by experienced assessors must be acknowledged. The 'halo effect', for example, which occurs because of forming first impressions, has been shown to provide accurate judgements although it reduces the opportunities in a particular rating for the student to demonstrate proficiency and causes difficulty in providing feedback on strengths and weaknesses (Wood 2014). Although with training, leniency and halo errors are reduced, it could be accompanied by less accurate measures.

Rater assessment is a complex process, and attempts have been made to study rater cognition. Further research in this area is needed to understand the cognitive processes that determine how and why raters vary in their assessment and scoring of student performances.

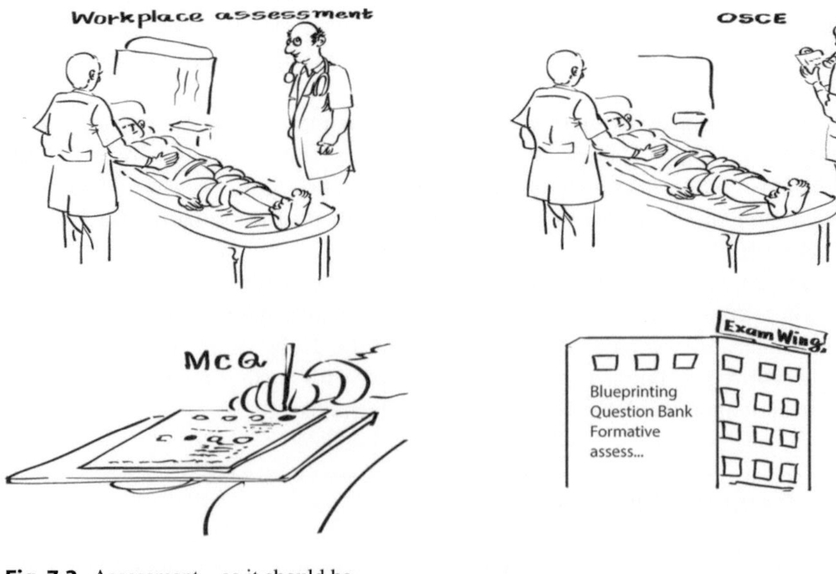

Fig. 7.3 Assessment—as it should be

Conclusions

There is an increasing awareness that the primary role of assessment is to help learning. This has brought about a move away from the practice of a single summing up of a student's achievement in the training programme to having a planned continuous programme of the student's progress in the course. Such a programmatic approach is important to address all aspects of competence expected in a graduate doctor, some of which are better assessed longitudinally. While acknowledging the importance of high-stakes examination for determining qualification, classroom assessments designed by the teacher play a significant role in ensuring a high quality of the learning experience. In the high-stakes setting which serves the purpose of certification of competence, defensible assessments need to be implemented with attention to metrics and post-examination analysis to optimize the process.

References

Archer JC (2010) State of the science in health professional education: effective feedback: effective feedback in health professional education. Med Educ 44:101–108. https://doi.org/10.1111/j.1365-2923.2009.03546.x

Baghdady M, Carnahan H, Lam EWN, Woods NN (2014) Test-enhanced learning and its effect on comprehension and diagnostic accuracy. Med Educ 48:181–188. https://doi.org/10.1111/medu.12302

Black P, Wiliam D (2009) Developing the theory of formative assessment. Educ Assess Eval Account 21:5–31. https://doi.org/10.1007/s11092-008-9068-5

Black P, Wiliam D (2010) Inside the black box: raising standards through classroom assessment. Phi Delta Kappan 92:81–90

Borsboom D, Mellenbergh GJ, van Heerden J (2004) The concept of validity. Psychol Rev 111:1061–1071. https://doi.org/10.1037/0033-295X.111.4.1061

Braun H, Kanjee A, Bettinger E, Kremer M (2006) Improving education through assessment, innovation, and evaluation. American Academy of Arts and Sciences, Cambridge, MA

Case SM, Swanson DB, Becker DF (1996) Verbosity, window dressing, and red herrings: do they make a better test item? Acad Med 71:S28–S30

Case SM, Swanson DB (2001) Constructing written test questions for the basic and clinical sciences. National Board of Medical Examiners, Philadelphia. Available from http://www.medbev.umontreal.ca/docimo/DocSource/NBME_MCQ.pdf

Charlin B, Brailovsky C, Leduc C, Blouin D (1998) The diagnosis script questionnaire: a new tool to assess a specific dimension of clinical competence. Adv Health Sci Educ 3:51–58

Cilliers FJ, Schuwirth LWT, Herman N, Adendorff HJ, van der Vleuten CPM (2012) A model of the pre-assessment learning effects of summative assessment in medical education. Adv Health Sci Educ 17:39–53. https://doi.org/10.1007/s10459-011-9292-5

Cook DA, Brydges R, Ginsburg S, Hatala R (2015) A contemporary approach to validity arguments: a practical guide to Kane's framework. Med Educ 49:560–575. https://doi.org/10.1111/medu.12678

Crooks TJ (1988) The impact of classroom evaluation practices on students. Rev Educ Res 58:438–481

Dannefer EF, Henson LC (2007) The portfolio approach to competency-based assessment at the Cleveland Clinic Lerner College of Medicine. Acad Med 82:493–502

van der Pol J, van den Berg BAM, Admiraal WF, Simons PRJ (2008) The nature, reception, and use of online peer feedback in higher education. Comput Educ 51:1804–1817. https://doi.org/10.1016/j.compedu.2008.06.001

van der Vleuten CPM, Schuwirth LWT (2005) Assessing professional competence: from methods to programmes. Med Educ 39:309–317. https://doi.org/10.1111/j.1365-2929.2005.02094.x
van der Vleuten CPM, Heeneman S, Schuwirth LWT (2017) Programmatic assessment. In: Dent JA, Harden RM, Hunt D (eds) A practical guide for medical teachers, 5th edn. Elsevier, Edinburgh, pp 295–303
Dijkstra J, Van der Vleuten CPM, Schuwirth LWT (2010) A new framework for designing programmes of assessment. Adv Health Sci Educ 15:379–393. https://doi.org/10.1007/s10459-009-9205-z
Downing SM (2003) Validity: on the meaningful interpretation of assessment data. Med Educ 37:830–837
Downing SM (2004) Reliability: on the reproducibility of assessment data. Med Educ 38:1006–1012
Dudek NL, Marks MB, Regehr G (2005) Failure to fail: the perspectives of clinical supervisors. Acad Med 80:S84–S87
Evans C (2013) Making sense of assessment feedback in higher education. Rev Educ Res 83:70–120. https://doi.org/10.3102/0034654312474350
Friedman Ben-David MF (2000) AMEE Guide No. 18: standard setting in student assessment. Med Teach 22:120–130. https://doi.org/10.1080/01421590078526
Gierl MJ, Lai H, Turner SR (2012) Using automatic item generation to create multiple-choice test items: automatic generation of test items. Med Educ 46:757–765. https://doi.org/10.1111/j.1365-2923.2012.04289.x
Gleeson F (1997) AMEE Medical Education Guide No. 9. Assessment of clinical competence using the Objective Structured Long Examination Record (OSLER). Med Teach 19:7–14. https://doi.org/10.3109/01421599709019339
Green ML, Holmboe E (2010) Perspective: the ACGME toolbox: half empty or half full? Acad Med 85:787–790
Harden RM, Gleeson FA (1979) Assessment of clinical competence using an objective structured clinical examination (OSCE). Med Educ 13:41–54
Hattie J, Timperley H (2007) The power of feedback. Rev Educ Res 77:81–112. https://doi.org/10.3102/003465430298487
Hejri SM, Jalili M (2014) Standard setting in medical education: fundamental concepts and emerging challenges. Med J Islam Repub Iran 28:34
Hift RJ (2014) Should essays and other "open-ended"-type questions retain a place in written summative assessment in clinical medicine? BMC Med Educ 14:249
Jonsson A, Svingby G (2007) The use of scoring rubrics: reliability, validity and educational consequences. Educ Res Rev 2:130–144. https://doi.org/10.1016/j.edurev.2007.05.002
Kane M (2009) Validating the interpretations and uses of test scores. In: Lissitz RW (ed) The concept of validity: revisions, new directions and applications. IAP, Charlotte, NC, pp 39–64
Kane M (2012) Validating score interpretations and uses. Lang Test 29:3–17
Kang SHK, McDermott KB, Roediger HL (2007) Test format and corrective feedback modify the effect of testing on long-term retention. Eur J Cogn Psychol 19:528–558. https://doi.org/10.1080/09541440601056620
Karpicke JD, Roediger HL (2008) The critical importance of retrieval for learning. Science 319:966–968
Kerdijk W, Cohen-Schotanus J, Mulder BF, Muntinghe FLH, Tio RA (2015) Cumulative versus end-of-course assessment: effects on self-study time and test performance. Med Educ 49:709–716. https://doi.org/10.1111/medu.12756
Kromann CB, Bohnstedt C, Jensen ML, Ringsted C (2010) The testing effect on skills learning might last 6 months. Adv Health Sci Educ 15:395–401. https://doi.org/10.1007/s10459-009-9207-x
Lew SR, Page GG, Schuwirth LW, Baron-Maldonado M, Lescop JM, Paget NS, J Southgate L, Wade WB (2002) Procedures for establishing defensible programmes for assessing practice performance. Med Educ 36:936–941
Lubarsky S, Dory V, Duggan P, Gagnon R, Charlin B (2013) Script concordance testing: from theory to practice: AMEE Guide No. 75. Med Teach 35:184–193. https://doi.org/10.3109/0142159X.2013.760036

MacLellan E (2001) Assessment for learning: the differing perceptions of tutors and students. Assess & Eval High Educ 26:307–318. https://doi.org/10.1080/02602930120063466
McKinley DW, Norcini JJ (2014) Standard setting for performance based examinations – AMEE Guide No. 85. Med Teach 36:97–110
Miller GE (1990) Assessment of clinical skills/competence/performance. Acad Med 65:S63–S67
Mislevy RJ, Steinberg LS, Almond RG (2003) Focus article: on the structure of educational assessments. Measurement (Mahwah, N J) 1:3–62. https://doi.org/10.1207/S15366359MEA0101_02
Nelson MM, Schunn CD (2009) The nature of feedback: how different types of peer feedback affect writing performance. Instr Sci 37:375–401. https://doi.org/10.1007/s11251-008-9053-x
Newton PE (2007) Clarifying the purposes of educational assessment. Assess Educ Princ Pol Pract 14(2):149–170. https://doi.org/10.1080/09695940701478321
Norcini JJ (2002) The death of the long case? BMJ 324:408–409
Norcini J, Burch V (2007) Workplace-based assessment as an educational tool: AMEE Guide No. 31. Med Teach 29(9):855–871
Page G (1999). Writing key features problems for the clinical reasoning skills examination. Accessed from http://www.idealmed.org/workshop/SectionD-KeyFeatures.pdf
Page G, Bordage G, Allen T (1995) Developing key feature problems and examinations to assess clinical decision-making skills. Acad Med 70:194–201
Pell G, Homer MS, Roberts TE (2008) Assessor training: its effects on criterion-based assessment in a medical context. Int J Res Meth Educ 31:143–154. https://doi.org/10.1080/17437270802124525
Pell G, Fuller R, Homer M, Roberts T (2010) How to measure the quality of the OSCE: a review of metrics – AMEE guide no. 49. Med Teach 32:802–811
Peters H, Holzhausen Y, Boscardin C, ten Cate O, Chen HC (2017) Twelve tips for the implementation of EPAs for assessment and entrustment decisions. Med Teach 39:802–807. https://doi.org/10.1080/0142159X.2017.1331031
Pugh D, Regehr G (2016) Taking the sting out of assessment: is there a role for progress testing? Med Educ 50:721–729. https://doi.org/10.1111/medu.12985
Quantrill SJ, Tun JK (2012) Workplace-based assessment as an educational tool. Guide supplement 31.5 – viewpoint. Med Teach 34:417–418. https://doi.org/10.3109/0142159X.2012.668234
Ramaprasad A (1983) On the definition of feedback. Behav Sci 28:4–13. https://doi.org/10.1002/bs.3830280103
Reiner CM, Bothell TW, Sudweeks RR, Wood B (2002) Preparing effective essay questions: a self-directed workbook for educators. New Forums Press. Accessed from https://testing.byu.edu/handbooks/WritingEffectiveEssayQuestions.pdf
Sadler DR (1989) Formative assessment and the design of instructional systems. Instr Sci 18:119–144
Sadler DR (1998) Formative assessment: revisiting the territory. Assess Educ Princ Pol Pract 5(1):77–84. https://doi.org/10.1080/0969595980050104
Schleicher I, Leitner K, Juenger J, Moeltner A, Ruesseler M, Bender B, Sterz J, Schuettler K-F, Koenig S, Kreuder JG (2017) Examiner effect on the objective structured clinical exam – a study at five medical schools. BMC Med Educ 17. https://doi.org/10.1186/s12909-017-0908-1
Schuwirth LWT, van der Vleuten CPM (2004) Different written assessment methods: what can be said about their strengths and weaknesses? Med Educ 38:974–979. https://doi.org/10.1111/j.1365-2929.2004.01916.x
Schuwirth LWT, Van der Vleuten CPM (2011) Programmatic assessment: from assessment of learning to assessment for learning. Med Teach 33:478–485. https://doi.org/10.3109/0142159X.2011.565828
Stobart G (2012) Validity in formative assessment. In: Gardner J (ed) Assessment and learning, 2nd edn. SAGE Publications, Great Britain, pp 239–249
St-Onge C, Young M, Eva KW, Hodges B (2017) Validity: one word with a plurality of meanings. Adv Health Sci Educ 22:853–867. https://doi.org/10.1007/s10459-016-9716-3
Swanson DB, Case SM (1997) Assessment in basic science instruction: directions for practice and research. Adv Health Sci Educ 2:71–84
Tavakol M, Dennick R (2011) Post-examination analysis of objective tests. Med Teach 33:447–458. https://doi.org/10.3109/0142159X.2011.564682

Tavakol M, Dennick R (2012) Post-examination interpretation of objective test data: monitoring and improving the quality of high-stakes examinations: AMEE Guide No. 66. Med Teach 34:e161–e175. https://doi.org/10.3109/0142159X.2012.651178

Tavakol M, Dennick R (2017) The foundations of measurement and assessment in medical education. Med Teach 39:1010–1015. https://doi.org/10.1080/0142159X.2017.1359521

Tavares W, Eva KW (2013) Exploring the impact of mental workload on rater-based assessments. Adv Health Sci Educ 18:291–303. https://doi.org/10.1007/s10459-012-9370-3

Tio RA, Schutte B, Meiboom AA, Greidanus J, Dubois EA, Bremers AJA, the Dutch Working Group of the Interuniversity Progress Test of Medicine (2016) The progress test of medicine: the Dutch experience. Perspect Med Educ 5:51–55. https://doi.org/10.1007/s40037-015-0237-1

Trochim WMK (2007) The research methods knowledge base. Accessed from http://trochim.human.cornell.edu/kb/index.htm

Van Der Vleuten CP (1996) The assessment of professional competence: developments, research and practical implications. Adv Health Sci Educ 1:41–67

Wass V, Van der Vleuten C, Shatzer J, Jones R (2001) Assessment of clinical competence. Lancet 357:945–949

Wood TJ (2014) Exploring the role of first impressions in rater-based assessments. Adv Health Sci Educ 19:409–427. https://doi.org/10.1007/s10459-013-9453-9

Yorke M (2005) Formative assessment in higher education: its significance for employability, and steps towards its enhancement. Tert Educ Manag 11:219–238. https://doi.org/10.1080/13583883.2005.9967148

A Practical Approach

8

Objectives

1. Describe the practical approach to improve discipline-based undergraduate medical curriculum.
2. List the limitations of discipline-based undergraduate medical curriculum, and discuss relevant educational strategies to overcome them.

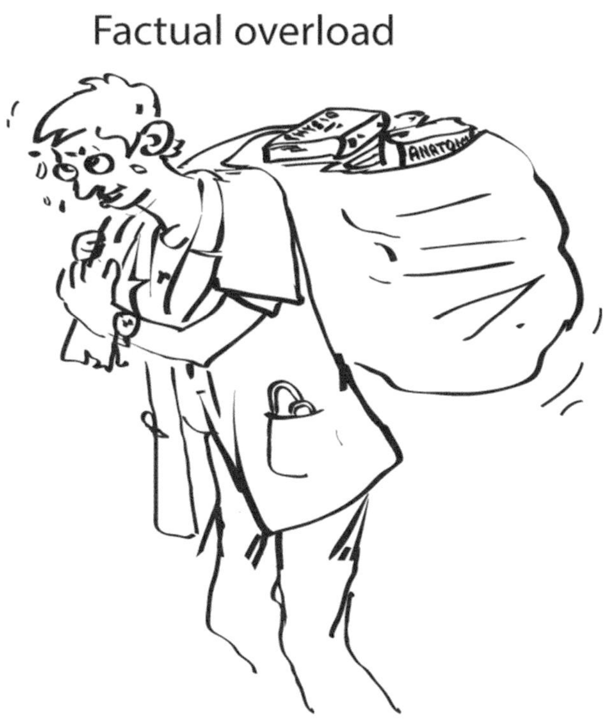

Fig. 8.1 Factual overload in curriculum

Kadambari D et al., *Improving Discipline-Based Undergraduate Medical Curriculum*, https://doi.org/10.1007/978-981-13-1310-3_8

8.1 Introduction

In the chapter 'Basics of Curriculum and Curriculum Change', implementation challenges, obstacles and facilitators of curriculum change are described. That chapter also describes cyclical problem-solving research-based approach to curriculum change and continuous improvement of undergraduate medical curriculum which involve making small changes on a regular basis. An appraisal of discipline-based undergraduate medical curriculum is done in the chapter 'Appraising Curriculum', and its generic strengths and limitations are described. The generic strengths of discipline-based undergraduate medical curriculum include the following:

(a) Existing discipline-based departmental organization.
(b) Teaching of fundamentals of disciplines by subject experts.

The generic limitations of discipline-based undergraduate medical curriculum are listed below:

(a) Factual information overload.
(b) Isolated learning and assessment.
(c) Teacher-centred approach.
(d) Opportunistic clinical teaching-learning.
(e) Neglect of MBBS programme goals.
(f) Resistance to change.

This chapter describes a practical approach to improve discipline-based undergraduate medical curriculum which involves retaining its strengths and overcoming its limitations by making small changes on a regular basis according to local situation.

8.2 A Practical Approach to Improve Discipline-Based Undergraduate Medical Curriculum

The basic principle is to retain the strengths of discipline-based undergraduate medical curriculum and to overcome its limitations by using educational strategies which are supported by evidence in literature. As the extent of limitations of discipline-based undergraduate medical curriculum may vary in different medical schools, the extent of various educational strategies needed may also vary in different medical schools. Furthermore, different medical schools may likely to overcome different limitations or different sets of limitations at different times. A cyclical problem-solving research-based approach to curriculum change is to be used for continuous improvement of undergraduate medical curriculum. Small changes are made on a regular basis. Curriculum change needs a curriculum committee to plan and implement curriculum changes and to evaluate the changes.

8.3 Retaining Strengths of Discipline-Based Undergraduate Medical Curriculum

Discipline-based undergraduate medical curriculum has the generic strengths of existing discipline-based departmental organization and teaching of fundamentals of disciplines by subject experts. These strengths are retained.

8.4 Overcoming Limitations of Discipline-Based Undergraduate Medical Curriculum

The limitations of discipline-based undergraduate medical curriculum and educational strategies suggested in literature to overcome them are given in Table 8.1.

The basics of generic educational strategies to overcome limitations of discipline-based undergraduate medical curriculum are described with supporting evidence from literature.

8.4.1 Core Curriculum with Options

The World Summit on Medical Education (World Federation for Medical Education 1993) and Tomorrow's Doctors (General Medical Council 1993) recommended core curriculum with options in response to the problem of factual information overload. However, core curriculum with options emerged as an important strategy of curriculum planning and was recognized in 1990s as a major step forward in medical education (Harden and Davis 1995). Core curriculum clearly defines the essential knowledge, skills and attitudes which are to be mastered by all students for maintaining the standards (Harden and Davis 1995). Perceptions of core curriculum included core as essentials of a discipline and core as essential competencies for clinical practice (Harden and Davis 1995). Harden and Davis (1995) described seven Cs, certification, capability, comprehensiveness, consistency, constructivism, choice and compacted curriculum, as the philosophical basis of core curriculum. Core curriculum can define competencies needed for a medical graduate which can

Table 8.1 Limitations of discipline-based undergraduate medical curriculum and educational strategies to overcome them

Limitations	Educational strategies
(a) Factual information overload	1. Core curriculum with options
(b) Isolated learning and assessment	2. Integrated learning
(c) Teacher-centred approach	3. Student-centred approach
(d) Opportunistic clinical teaching-learning	4. Clinical presentation-based curriculum approach
	5. Entrustable professional activities
(e) Neglect of MBBS programme goals	6. Outcome-based education/competency-based education
(f) Resistance to change	7. Curriculum committee

be used for certification as a response to public expectation and demand for demonstrating relevance and accountability in medical education. Focus on competencies meets the expectation of the concept of education for capability. Comprehensiveness can be ensured by inclusion of all essential aspects in curriculum. Defining core curriculum ensures that there is consistency or uniformity in certification. Defining core content of core curriculum avoids factual information overload and facilitates deep understanding as part of constructivism. Core curriculum should take up only two-thirds of the curricular time (General Medical Council 1993). Thus one third of the curricular time can be used for study of options as per the choice of students. Students who can master the core curriculum in shorter time (compacted curriculum) can use longer time in studying options.

Core content of the core curriculum can be defined by agreeing to a list of clinical presentations and then agreeing on the requirements of basic science, behavioural science and clinical science for each presentation (Newble et al. 2005).

Options were called special study modules in the first edition of Tomorrow's Doctors (General Medical Council 1993) and student-selected components in the second edition of Tomorrow's Doctors (General Medical Council 2003). Special study modules are formal courses in which topics can be from the core curriculum for in-depth learning, from non-core medicine or from non-medical subjects (Harden and Davis 1995). Special study modules are chosen from a list given by faculty. Electives are chosen by students and are less formal for research or visit to a healthcare facility in another country (Harden and Davis 1995). The purpose of options is to give the student an opportunity to learn in an area of his or her interest.

8.4.2 Integrated Learning

In a discipline-based undergraduate medical curriculum/programme, students need to perform two tasks. They have to integrate knowledge from basic, behavioural and clinical sciences and then they have to apply the integrated scientific knowledge to solve patient problems. These tasks are not automatic. Students have to integrate what they learn separately. Integrated learning by students can be facilitated by using integration as an educational strategy. Integration as a strategy has been universally recommended in undergraduate medical curriculum (General Medical Council 1993; Medical Council of India 1997, 2012).

Harden (2000) has described the integration ladder as a continuum of 11 steps. These steps include isolation, awareness, harmonization, nesting, temporal coordination, sharing, correlation, complementary, multidisciplinary, interdisciplinary and transdisciplinary. Step 1 or isolation occurs in traditional discipline-based curriculum in which disciplines are taught in isolation independent of other disciplines. Steps 2–5 of integration do not involve joint teaching. In step 2 of awareness, disciplines share information about their objectives, content, topics and handouts. In step 3 of harmonization, there is mutual consultation between disciplines for planning. Step 4 of nesting involves inclusion of content (e.g. images) from other disciplines.

Step 5 of temporal coordination involves adjustment of scheduling so different aspects of same topic are covered at the same time in different disciplines. Temporal coordination can be system-based so same systems are taught in different disciplines at the same time facilitating integrated learning.

Steps 6–9 of integration involve joint teaching. In step 6 or sharing, there is joint teaching of common areas. Step 7 or correlation may include integrated sessions oriented to solve patient problems. In step 8 or complementary integration, equal time is given for discipline-based, and integrated teaching and assessment are both discipline-based and integrated. In step 9 or multidisciplinary integration, more time is given to integrated teaching (organized around systems or themes) than discipline-based teaching, there is integrated assessment and the identities of disciplines are maintained.

In step 10 or interdisciplinary integration, the disciplines are not identified, and programme is organized around themes, e.g. stages of life cycle. Step 11 or trans-disciplinary integration involves real-life learning. Clinical presentations can be used for organizing clinical learning during clinical postings (Harden 2000; Harden et al. 2000). There is integrated learning around clinical presentations which may be common between disciplines (e.g. abdominal pain), and there is problem-oriented learning which is context based. Learning is active and led by students under the guidance of teachers.

Learning objectives of patient contact in the first year commonly include 'understanding the patient experience and perspective of disease and health care' and 'understanding the social context of illness: the social determinants of health and the impact of disease on families and society' (Hopayian et al. 2007). Other learning objective of patient contact in first year can be to relate basic sciences to clinical presentations. Active observation using checklists and rating forms is better than passive observation in early clinical exposure (Kachur 2003). All patient-contact sessions should be preceded by preparation and followed by debriefing.

8.4.3 Student-Centred Approach

Student-centred approach implies ensuring high student engagement and use of constructivist approach by students for learning with understanding. Lectures should not exceed one third of the curricular time (Medical Council of India 1997, 2012). Modern methods such as audience response system (Nelson et al. 2012) can be used during lectures for ensuring student engagement. Team-based learning (Parmelee et al. 2013) is a new method which ensures student engagement. Group discussion, seminar and tutorial should be used more often (Medical Council of India 1997, 2012). Objective structured clinical examination and objective structured practical examination should be included in clinical teaching-learning and practical teaching-learning, respectively. Individual learning methods such as assignment, project, oral presentation, e-learning, skill lab learning and portfolio ensure student engagement and can be used with guidance and support.

8.4.4 Clinical Presentation-Based Curriculum Approach

In discipline-based approach to curriculum, content is organized around disciplines and controlled by departments (Papa and Harasym 1999). In clinical presentation-based curriculum approach, content is organized around clinical presentations and controlled by curriculum committee (Papa and Harasym 1999). Clinical presentation-based curriculum is an example of competency-based curriculum (Mandin et al. 1995). A clinical presentation is a common and important problem with which a patient presents to a doctor and which a medical graduate is expected to manage (Mandin et al. 1995). A clinical presentation is usually a symptom or symptom complex and less commonly a sign or laboratory/imaging result. The human body responds in a limited number of ways to an unlimited number of insults (Mandin et al. 1995). The Faculty of Medicine at the University of Calgary decided on a list of 120 clinical presentations (Mandin et al. 1995). Whatever knowledge was thought to be required to understand, diagnose and manage the clinical presentations and their common and important causal conditions constituted core knowledge (Mandin and Dauphinee 2000). A similar approach to decide core content has also been recommended by others (Cholerton and Jordan 2009; Leinster 2013). Some numbers of clinical presentations/problems used by others have been 87 (Ozkan et al. 2006), 94 (Newble et al. 2005) and 113 (Harden et al. 2000). The General Medical Council (2015) included 'diagnose and mange clinical presentations' as one outcome under the role of 'The doctor as a practitioner'. Pathways Curriculum of Harvard Medical School (2015) included 'ability to diagnose clinical problems' and 'solve clinical problems using medical knowledge and scientific evidence' as two of ten fundamental skills later renamed as Clinical Education Entrustable Professional Activities. Diagnosing and managing patient problems have been two objectives in undergraduate medical curriculum of Jawaharlal Institute of Postgraduate Medical Education and Research, Puducherry (Srinivasa 1995), and Medical Council of India's Regulations on Graduate Medical Education (1997) and a competency in Medical Council of India's Regulations on Graduate Medical Education—Proposed (2012).

Organization of clinical learning around clinical presentations has the advantages of problem-oriented and context-based learning and transdisciplinary integration (Harden 2000; Harden et al. 2000). Emphasis on clinical presentations can improve the process of data collection from patients, diagnostic process and primary care and bring much needed patient-centredness into medical practice. If core knowledge based on common and important clinical presentations and causal conditions is used for learning theoretical basis, its application to clinical problem-solving will be facilitated due to problem orientation and context basis.

8.4.5 Entrustable Professional Activities

An entrustable professional activity (EPA) is 'a unit of professional practice that can be fully entrusted to a trainee, as soon as he or she has demonstrated the necessary competence to execute this activity unsupervised' (ten Cate et al. 2015). EPAs are needed to implement competency-based education because competencies are personal qualities and need professional activities to demonstrate them. EPA-competency matrix is used to know which competencies are needed for a particular EPA (ten Cate et al. 2015). In postgraduate medical education, EPAs have been identified in many specialities (ten Cate et al. 2015). In undergraduate medical education, 'Core Entrustable Professional Activities for Entering Residency' including 13 EPAs have been proposed by the Association of American Medical Colleges (2014). 'AFMC Entrustable Professional Activities for the Transition from Medical School to Residency' including 12 EPAs have been identified by the Association of Faculties of Medicine of Canada (2016). Two of the 12 EPAs are included to 'obtain a history and perform a physical examination adapted to the patient's clinical situation' and 'formulate and justify a prioritized differential diagnosis'.

8.4.6 Outcome-Based Education/Competency-Based Education

It is universally agreed that as a part of social accountability, graduating doctors at the end of undergraduate medical educational programme should possess certain desirable abilities. These exit abilities are commonly expressed as outcomes or competencies. Thus we have the General Medical Council (UK) outcomes under three roles of the doctor as a scholar and a scientist, as a practitioner and as a professional (General Medical Council 2015) and the Scottish Doctor learning outcomes as part of a three-circle model of 'what the doctor is able to do', 'how the doctor approaches his/her practice' and 'the doctor as professional' (Scottish Deans' Medical Education Group 2018). We also have the Accreditation Council for Graduate Medical Education or ACGME (USA) competencies under the categories of patient care and procedural skills, medical knowledge, practice-based learning and improvement, interpersonal and communication skills, professionalism and system-based practice (Accreditation Council for Graduate Medical Education 2017) and the CanMEDS Physician Competency Framework (Canada) including the roles of medical expert, communicator, collaborator, leader, health advocate, scholar and professional (Frank et al. 2015).

The purpose of outcome-based education is to ensure that graduating doctors achieve desirable learning outcomes at the end of undergraduate medical educational programme. In outcome-based education, learning outcomes are identified, and these learning outcomes determine the content, learning process, assessment process and all other curricular issues (Harden et al. 1999). If learning outcomes are relevant to health needs of the society, outcome-based education ensures that the undergraduate medical educational curriculum/programme is aligned to societal health needs. Harden (2013) has described advantages of outcome-based education including attention to neglected areas of competence, tackling problem of information overload, assessment of learner's progress and continuation of education, student-centred and individual learning and accountability. Primacy of learning outcomes ensures that areas of competence such as communication and professionalism which are neglected in discipline-based curriculum are included in outcome-based curriculum. As learning outcomes decide the content, the problem of factual information overload can be controlled in outcome-based curriculum. As same learning outcomes with increasing levels of complexity can be used throughout undergraduate and postgraduate educational programmes, learning outcomes can be used for assessing learner's progress (Harden 2007). Clear expectations conveyed through learning outcomes promote self-learning by students. Availability of learning outcomes for undergraduate medical educational curriculum/programme and their certification provides evidence of relevance of programme as part of accountability to the society. Outcome-based education is a comprehensive strategy for undergraduate and postgraduate medical education. The limitation of outcome-based education is that it requires a curriculum committee for its management.

Outcome-based education can also be implemented in a stepwise manner starting with one role (medical expert) or two roles (medical expert and communicator) of the CanMEDS framework.

Competency is a type of outcome, and competency-based education is a type of outcome-based education. The main principles of competency-based education include focusing on outcomes, emphasizing abilities, de-emphasizing time-based training and promoting greater learner-centredness (Frank et al. 2010).

8.4.7 Curriculum Committee

The concept of curriculum committee is briefly described under central approach managing undergraduate curriculum in the chapter on Basics of Curriculum and Curriculum Change.

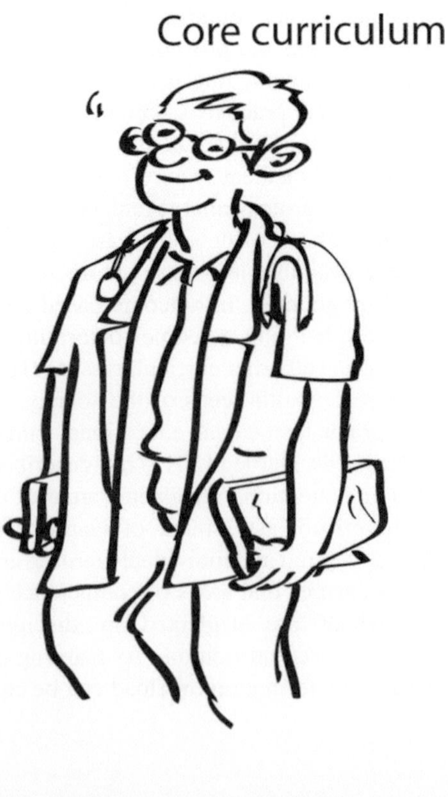

Fig. 8.2 Managing factual overload

Conclusions

The discipline-based undergraduate medical curriculum has strengths and limitations. The former are to be retained, and the latter are to be overcome using evidence-supported educational strategies. As the extent of limitations may vary in different medical schools, the extent of various educational strategies needed may also vary in different medical schools. In addition, different medical schools may like to tackle different limitations at different times. A cyclical problem-solving research-based approach to curriculum change is to be used for continuous improvement of undergraduate medical curriculum. Small changes are made on a regular basis. Curriculum committee is required for effective curriculum change.

References

Accreditation Council for Graduate Medical Education. ACGME (2017) Common programme requirements. Available from https://www.acgme.org/Portals/0/PFAssets/ProgramRequirements/CPRs_2017-07-01.pdf. Accessed 13 Jan 2018

Association of American Medical Colleges (2014) Core entrustable professional activities for entering residency. Curriculum developers' guide. Association of American Medical Colleges, Washington, DC Available from https://members.aamc.org/eweb/upload/core%20EPA%20Curriculum%20Dev%20Guide.pdf. Accessed 12 Jan 2018

Cholerton S, Jordan R (2009) Core curriculum and student-selected components. In: Dent JA, Harden RM (eds) A practical guide for medical teachers, 3rd edn. Churchill Livingstone Elsevier, Edinburgh, pp 193–201

Frank JR, Snell LS, ten Cate O, Holmboe ES, Carraccio C, Swing SR et al (2010) Competency-based medical education: theory to practice. Med Teach 32:638–645. PMID: 20662574. https://doi.org/10.3109/0142159X.2010.501190

Frank JR, Snell L, Sherbino J (eds) (2015) CanMEDS 2015 physician competency framework. Royal College of Physicians and Surgeons of Canada, Ottawa Available from www.royalcollege.ca/rcsite/documents/canmeds/canmeds-full-framework-e.pdf. Accessed 8 Jan 2018

General Medical Council (1993) Tomorrow's Doctors. Recommendations on undergraduate medical education, Dec 1993

General Medical Council (2003) Tomorrow's Doctors

General Medical Council (2015) Outcomes for graduates (Tomorrow's Doctors), July 2015. Available from https://www.gmc-uk.org/Outcomes_for_graduates_Jul_15_1216.pdf_61408029.pdf. Accessed 8 Jan 2018

Harden RM (2000) The integration ladder: a tool for curriculum planning and evaluation. Med Educ 34:551–557. https://doi.org/10.1046/j.1365-2923.2000.00697.x

Harden RM (2007) Learning outcomes as a tool to assess progression. Med Teach 29:678–682. PMID: 18236255. https://doi.org/10.1080/01421590701729955

Harden RM (2013) Outcome-based education. In: Dent JA, Harden RM (eds) A practical guide for medical teachers, 4th edn. Churchill Livingstone Elsevier, London, pp 151–156

Harden RM, Davis MH (1995) AMEE Medical Education Guide No. 5. The core curriculum with options or special study modules. Med Teach 17(2):125–148 Available from https://amee.org/getattachment/AMEE-Initiatives/ESME-Courses/AMEE-ESME-Face-to-Face-Courses/ESME/ESME-Online-Resources-China-Dec-2015/AMEE-Guide-No-5.PDF. Accessed 12 Jan 2018

Harden RM, Crosby JR, Davis MH (1999) AMEE Guide No.14: outcome-based education: Part 1 – An introduction to outcome-based education. Med Teach 21(1):7–14. https://doi.org/10.1080/01421599979969

Harden RM, Crosby F, Davis MH, Howie PW, Struthers AD (2000) Task-based learning: the answer to integration and problem-based learning in the clinical years. Med Educ 34:391–397 PMID: 10760125. Available from http://citeseerx.ist.psu.edu/viewdoc/download?doi=10.1.1.462.8610&rep=rep1&type=pdf. Accessed 12 Jan 2018

Harvard Medical School (2015) Pathways curriculum. Available from https://hms.harvard.edu/sites/default/files/assets/Sites/PME/files/Design%20Team%20Summaries%2011.13.15%20Final.pdf. Accessed 12 Jan 2018

Hopayian K, Howe A, Dagley V (2007) A survey of UK medical schools' arrangements for early patient contact. Med Teach 29:806–813. https://doi.org/10.1080/01421590701543125

Kachur EK (2003) Observation during early clinical exposure—an effective instructional tool or a bore? Med Educ 37:88–89. https://doi.org/10.1046/j.1365-2923.2003.01421.x

Leinster S (2013) The undergraduate curriculum and clinical teaching in the early years. In: Dent JA, Harden RM (eds) A practical guide for medical teachers, 4th edn. Churchill Livingstone Elsevier, London, pp 16–22

Mandin H, Dauphinee WD (2000) Conceptual guidelines for developing and maintaining curriculum and examination objectives: the experience of the Medical Council of Canada. Acad Med 75(10):1031–1037 Available from http://journals.lww.com/academicmedicine/Abstract/2000/10000/Conceptual_Guidelines_for_Developing_and.24.aspx. Accessed 12 Jan 2018

Mandin H, Harasym P, Eagle C, Watanabe M (1995) Developing a "Clinical Presentation" curriculum at the University of Calgary. Acad Med 70(3):186–193 http://journals.lww.com/academicmedicine/pages/default.aspx

Medical Council of India (1997) Regulations on graduate medical education. Available from https://www.mciindia.org/documents/rulesAndRegulations/GME_REGULATIONS.pdf. Accessed 8 Jan 2018

Medical Council of India (2012) Regulations on graduate medical education – proposed. Available from http://iafmonline.in/data/circular-notifications/Revised-GME-2012.pdf. Accessed 8 Jan 2018

ten Cate O, Chen HC, Hoff RG, Peters H, Bok H, Van der Schaaf M (2015) Curriculum development for the workplace using Entrustable Professional Activities (EPAs): AMEE Guide No. 99. Med Teach 37(11):983–1002. PMID: 26172347. https://doi.org/10.3109/0142159X.2015.1060308

Nelson C, Hartling L, Campbell S, Oswald AE (2012) The effects of audience response systems on learning outcomes in health professions education. A BEME systematic review: BEME Guide No. 21. Med Teach 34(6):e386–e405. PMID: 22578049. https://doi.org/10.3109/0142159X.2012.680938

Newble D, Stark P, Bax N, Lawson M (2005) Developing an outcome-focused core curriculum. Med Educ 39:680–687. PMID: 15960788. https://doi.org/10.1111/j.1365-2929.2005.02198.x

Ozkan H, Degirmenci B, Musal B, Itil O, Akalin E, Kilinc O, Ozkan S, Alici E (2006) Task-based learning programme for clinical years of medical education. Educ Health 19(1):32–42. PMID: 16531300. https://doi.org/10.1080/13576280500534826

Papa FJ, Harasym PH (1999) Medical curriculum reform in North America, 1765 to the present: a cognitive science perspective. Acad Med 74(2):154–164 PMID: 10065057. http://journals.lww.com/academicmedicine/pages/default.aspx

Parmelee D, Hudes P, Michaelsen LK (2013) Team-based learning. In: Dent JA, Harden RM (eds) A practical guide for medical teachers, 4h edn. Churchill Livingstone Elsevier, London, pp 173–182

Scottish Deans' Medical Education Group (2018) The Scottish Doctor. Learning outcomes for the medical undergraduate in Scotland: a foundation for competent and reflective practitioners, 3rd edn. Association for Medical Education in Europe (AMEE), Dundee Available from http://www.scottishdoctor.org/resources/scotdoc3.pdf. Accessed 12 Jan 2018

Srinivasa DK (1995) Curriculum planning. In: Ananthakrishnan N, Sethuraman KR, Kumar S (eds) Medical education: principles and practice. National Teacher Training Centre, JIPMER, Pondicherry, pp 165–173

The AFMC EPA Working Group (2016) AFMC entrustable professional activities for the transition from Medical School to Residency. Association of Faculties of Medicine of Canada; September 2016. Available from https://afmc.ca/sites/default/files/documents/AFMC_Entrustable_Professional_Activities_EN_0.pdf. Accessed 12 Jan 2018

World Federation for Medical Education (1993) Proceedings of the World Summit On Medical Education. Walton HJ (Ed.). Med Educ 28(Suppl 1):140–149

Part IV

Support Systems for Planning and Implementing an Improved Curriculum

9 Leadership in Medical Education

Objectives

1. To understand the concept of curricular leadership.
2. To explain the need for curricular leadership in medical education.
3. To enumerate the functions of curriculum leadership.
4. To appreciate the importance of curricular leadership in institution building.

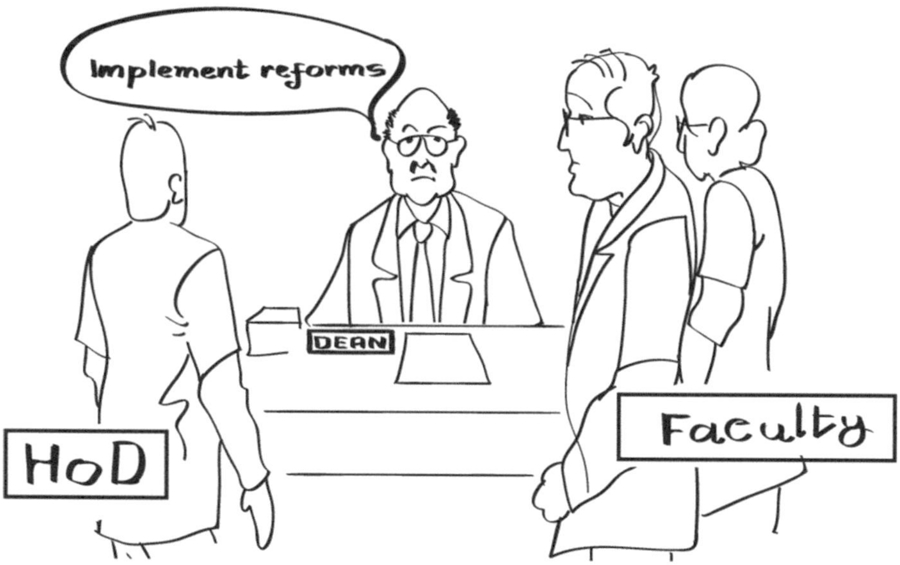

Fig. 9.1 Leadership: autocratic

Kadambari D et al., *Improving Discipline-Based Undergraduate Medical Curriculum*, https://doi.org/10.1007/978-981-13-1310-3_9

9.1 Who Are Leading Our Medical Schools?

It is a convention that people who have gone all walks of medical professional life leads a medical school in India. Their experience ranges from senior residency, tutorship, lectureship, assistant professor, associate professor and professor, head of the units, head of departments and officer in charge of various sections. The experience gained through this career ladder may or may not have prepared the leader fully to lead a medical school. It all depends on his exposure and contribution to the field that he has worked in. Sometimes leadership is forced upon someone who do not have interest or attitude towards leadership by virtue of their seniority or for certain political reasons (McCarthy 2002).

9.2 Challenges and Issues in Medical Education

The Indian medical education system is one of the oldest and largest in the world and is currently fast transforming from didactic classes to the concept of 'learning by doing' (Supe and Burdick 2006). Current transformation in medical education is mainly because of the rapidly changing global environment and expanding higher education. Increasing demands on the quality aspects of medical education has led to increasing complexity of the nature of medical education (Jacobson et al. 2015). Changing government policies and educational policy also have an influence on medical education. The role of nongovernment sectors has created both positive and negative impact on the delivery of medical education in India (Majumder et al. 2004). The changing needs and demands of multiple stakeholders have made medical education more vulnerable to criticisms. Medical education is expected to deliver high-quality student learning experience, enhance research outputs and ensure fitness for employment at all levels or for higher studies. The accreditation agencies use various metrics to identify and reward medical education institutions. The growing impact of technology on teaching-learning methods, assessment and evaluation in medical education and the expectations of funding agencies have raised the concerns about quality medical education (Chretien et al. 2014). Interprofessionalism is another area that poses challenges to make a physician work cordially in an interprofessional environment. All these have made the physicians to play a dynamic role, or their professional roles as physicians keep changing according to the needs of the healthcare system (Mette et al. 2016). This has initiated a paradigm shift of medical education and has made medical education a dynamic entity of this century (Till et al. 2017).

These changes in demands in the field of medical education pose new challenges for the educational leaders. In order to cope up with these challenges, the leaders have to be able to adapt to the societal needs and to be able to implement changes accordingly while also being responsive to the structural requirements of the academic organization, which is a challenge in itself. This brings in the context of need for effective leadership and leadership development in medical education. Best medical facilities and the various successful techniques of development of educational leadership have to be better understood, in order to fulfil this need. The need for leadership and political commitment to accomplish relevant, evidence-based medical education has been well emphasized in a government-commissioned report written by (Majumder et al. 2004).

9.3 The Concept of 'Curriculum' and 'Leadership'

There are many definitions and interpretations of curriculum. Bell and Baker (1997) interpreted the term curriculum in a broader sense by suggesting that the term can have multiple layers of meaning based on its type. They described these types as the *planned curriculum, taught curriculum, learned curriculum, assessed curriculum* and *hidden curriculum*. The *planned* curriculum is what the teacher plans and intends on teaching, while the *taught* curriculum is what actually happens during the course of the lesson where it tends to change under the influence of the students' ideas, questions and needs. The *learned* curriculum refers to 'what the students actually take away with them', which may or may not be the taught curriculum. The *assessed* curriculum is that which the teacher assesses, and it does not necessarily reflect all that the students have learnt. The last type of curriculum, i.e. the *hidden* curriculum, is the implicit and unintended learning which happens to take place in the classroom most of the time (Thompson et al. 2013).

There are two forms of leadership as discussed by a number of authors, and they are transactional and transformational leadership. Leithwood and Seashore-Louis (2011) suggest that the transactional leadership is based on the exchange of services controlled by the leader, whereas transformational leadership helps other people to improve in their practices. Transformational educational leaders are witnessed to be promoting a collaborative culture by encouraging group dynamics and teamwork, and they are also seen to be fostering the all-round development of the teachers. This form of leadership helps teachers change the instructional behaviour of the students, thus promoting leadership qualities in them.

Connelly et al. (2008) explained that the transformative curriculum leadership aims mainly on developing and implementing instructional interactions and educational programmes according to the interests of the students. The main idea behind transformative curriculum is to learn and grow by committing mistakes and is thus grounded in self and social examination (Langendyk et al. 2016; Quintero 2014). Blase and Blase (1999) cited that transformative curriculum leaders work to include multiple perspectives, encourage creative problem-solving and nurture critical thinking.

9.4 Concept of Curricular Leadership

Fidler (1997) points out that 'curricular leadership' is referred to as 'instructional leadership' in the United States, which makes the concept of curricular leadership conspicuous. He also says that the concept is to lead by instructing which means that the head of the institution must have an impact on the professional work done in the educational institution, such as teaching, learning and assessment activities.

Frich et al. (2015) state that there are two points of view in which instructional leadership can be considered, one being the functional approach and the other process approach. Sherrin (2000) says that the functional approach requires the leaders to define the school mission, manage curriculum and instruction, supervise teaching, monitor student progress and promote an instructional environment.

9.5 Why do Medical Colleges Need Curriculum Leaders?

If the purpose of medical colleges is to adequately prepare students for a professional life in a world that is becoming increasingly complex, then principals, teachers and other education professionals must constantly strive to provide the most relevant and up-to-date programmes they can. Sergiovanni (1996) suggests that the administrators, teachers, parents and students must accept and view leadership as an important moral obligation. Leadership is a shared responsibility for exercising and ensuring the leadership motto. Teachers alone are expected to be responsible for providing leadership in classrooms, but we must understand that leadership is a shared responsibility and must therefore be accepted by administrators and parents also. Together they can contribute to the provision and success of leadership. In order to achieve this, the principals and teachers must continue to develop their personal and professional knowledge, skills and understanding and must make the curriculum development an ongoing process. The use of curriculum leaders is one of the ways in which the ongoing professional development can be promoted. Hence, it can be reiterated that curriculum leadership provides:

1. Directions and clarity on what should every student know and be able to do with proper attitude in order to meet the national health goals. This also includes the qualities to be fostered among the medical graduates to fulfil the health needs of their society.
2. Opportunities to develop and empower future leaders by exposing the stakeholders like faculty, students and others to appropriate educational and professional environment and by entrusting them with curriculum and educational assignments.
3. Opportunity for continuous improvement by sensing the ongoing developments in medical education regularly and exploring the ways how successfully they can be implemented in their educational setup. The medical schools should consider themselves as a learning organization which continuously look for new avenues for growth and development to bring in quantitative and qualitative changes in medical education.
4. Opportunity to establish goals for the institution in accordance with the goals set by the national and international agencies. These goals provide teachers, students and stakeholders of education on what to aim for as part of their professional enterprise.
5. Opportunity for improved alignment. The intended curriculum is usually in the form of a document, the taught curriculum is the curriculum transacted across the professional years and learned curriculum is the curriculum that is assessed

to certify the students. One of the tasks of curriculum leadership is to use the right methods to bring the written, the taught, the supported and the tested curriculums into closer alignment, so that the learned curriculum is maximized.

9.6 Functions or Role of a Curriculum Leader in Medical Education

Frich et al. (2015) and Glatthorn (2000) wrote, 'One of the tasks of curriculum leadership is to use the right methods to bring the written, the taught, the supported, and the tested curriculums into closer alignment, so that the learned curriculum is maximized'. Advancements in education and educational technologies have changed the way the teachers teach and the way the students learn their subjects. Though more and more advances are taking place in education and educational technologies, there are no much takers especially from the teachers' side. A curriculum leader should be the one who can sense the recent advances in education and try incorporating in the existing system with the support of all the stakeholders (Langendyk et al. 2016). However, the findings from the literature review refer to the importance of the following facets of a curriculum leadership at both departmental and institutional levels:

- Providing direction and creating a structure to support the direction.
- Fostering a supportive and collaborative environment for progressive development and achievement of stated institutional goals.
- Establishing trustworthiness as a leader by demonstrating personal integrity and having credibility to act as a role model.
- Facilitating participation in decision-making at all levels of institutional activities.
- Ensuring proper communication about developments to all the stakeholders.
- Representing the department/institution to advance its cause(s) and networking on its behalf.
- Respecting existing culture while seeking to instil values through a vision for the department/institution.
- Ensuring and protecting autonomy of all staff.

The need for leader to create a harmonious environment and/or context for academics and others to fulfil their potential and interest in their work is seen at the heart of the above list. The significance of fostering a collegial climate of mutual supportiveness and the maintenance of autonomy is vital in the academic context.

9.7 Curriculum Leadership for 'Institution Building'

The term 'institution building' has been used to refer to both the process of an institution's internal development and to its ability to strengthen its impact upon the society. *Leadership for Institution Building in Education* (2006) states that the promotion of an institution's impact on the society can be attained by transforming the institution into an active part of a community in such a way that the institution gets to project new values and bring about changes in the community. Therefore, the management of an institution must pay attention to this aspect of institution building also. In the case of a medical college, the major function of management is to make the institution more effective as well as an efficient one. There are five main aspects with which the effectiveness of an institution can be conceived, and they are achievement of goals, development of people, expansion or growth, self-renewal and impact on the larger community. Every institution has its own defined goals, and the role of the management is to ensure that these goals are achieved quickly and with minimum effort. These goals may include providing education, doing research, preparing policies and strategies, evaluating programmes, supporting various projects, etc. Even though various criteria can be brought up to evaluate the cost and the extent of the achievement of these goals, the quantitative measurement of the effectiveness of these goals proves to be a difficult task. In certain cases, the impact of an institution can only be judged in the long term. It can also be said that it is not always possible to divide up and share the relative impact of an institution and of other sources. Management should without a doubt ensure both the qualitative aspects of achievement of goals and efficiency, in terms of input-output ratio. In addition to the achievement of its defined goals, an institution needs to be concerned with the growth of its own people as it is they that play different roles and work at various levels. An educational institution, particularly at the tertiary level, has to look after this important dimension. A staff's continuous professional growth and the undertaking of higher responsibilities in the institution are the main aspects that contribute to his/her development.

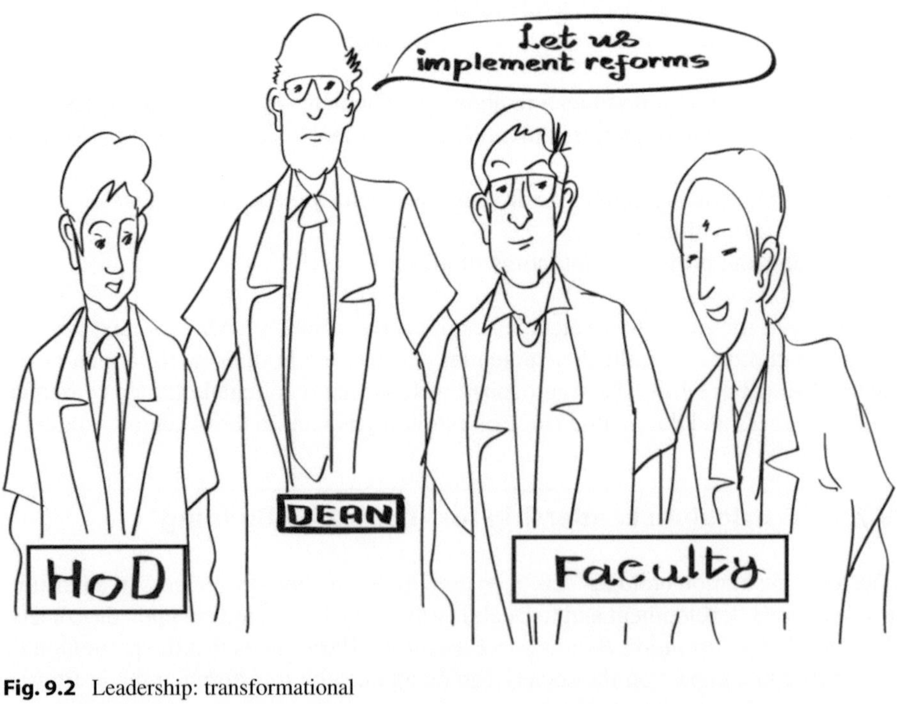

Fig. 9.2 Leadership: transformational

Conclusion

The most important understanding in the context of educational institution is that not all the people at the helm are born leaders. It cannot be expected of a vice-chancellor of a university or a principal of a college to lead his/her institution to glory and peaks of excellence all by himself/herself. Educational institutions are self-governing organizations and collegiality is the core of the relationship that binds its members. It is often in these kinds of environment in which the qualities of leadership are manifested. It should be remembered that it is not the person at the top alone who is the only leader, but that there is leadership at several levels. The positions of the pro-vice-chancellor, vice-chancellor, dean or departmental head are the few of the multiple levels of leadership that can be found in an institution; in fact at all levels, there is leadership, and it is the emergence of such leadership that makes an educational institution a dynamically evolving organization. The total sum of the contributions of the members is what is finally evaluated as the performance of the institution, i.e. the performance of the institution depends upon the performance of its members. When the members function in teams, they develop synergy which boosts up the level of productivity of each member of the group which cannot possibly be attained through individual contributions. It would therefore be beneficial if work in the institutions were organized around departments, interest groups or group projects. In this type of leadership, the leader develops a common interest among the team members by motivating them to strive towards a common goal.

References

Bell B, Baker R (1997) Curriculum development in science: policy-to-practice and practice-to-policy. In: Developing the science curriculum in Aotearoa, New Zealand. Longman, Auckland

Blase J, Blase J (1999) Principals' instructional leadership and teacher development: teachers' perspectives. Educ Adm Q 35:349–378. https://doi.org/10.1177/0013161X99353003

Chretien KC, Yarris LM, Lin M (2014) Technology in graduate medical education: shifting the paradigm and advancing the field. J Grad Med Educ 6:195–196. https://doi.org/10.4300/JGME-D-14-00157.1

Connelly FM, He MF, Phillion J (2008) The SAGE handbook of curriculum and instruction. SAGE, Los Angeles

Fidler B (1997) School leadership: some key ideas. Sch Leadersh Manag 17:23–38. https://doi.org/10.1080/13632439770140

Frich JC, Brewster AL, Cherlin EJ, Bradley EH (2015) Leadership development programs for physicians: a systematic review. J Gen Intern Med 30:656–674. https://doi.org/10.1007/s11606-014-3141-1

Glatthorn AA (2000) The principal as curriculum leader: shaping what is taught and tested, 2nd edn. Corwin Press, Inc., Thousand Oaks, CA

Jacobson S, McCarthy M, Pounder D (2015) What makes a leadership preparation program exemplary? J Res Leadersh Educ 10:63–76. https://doi.org/10.1177/1942775115569420

Langendyk V, Mason G, Wang S (2016) How do medical educators design a curriculum that facilitates student learning about professionalism? Int J Med Educ 7:32–43. https://doi.org/10.5116/ijme.5683.c2e0

Leadership for Institution Building in Education (2006) Icfai University Press, Hyderabad

Leithwood K, Seashore-Louis K (2011) Linking leadership to student learning. Jossey-Bass, an imprint of Wiley

Majumder AA, D'Souza U, Rahman S (2004) Trends in medical education: challenges and directions for need-based reforms of medical training in South-East Asia. Indian J Med Sci 58:369–380

McCarthy MM (2002) Educational leadership preparation programs: a glance at the past with an eye toward the future. Leadersh Policy Sch 1:201–221. https://doi.org/10.1076/lpos.1.3.201.7890

Mette M, Dölken M, Hinrichs J, Narciß E, Schüttpelz-Brauns K, Weihrauch U, Fritz HM (2016) Comprehension through cooperation: medical students and physiotherapy apprentices learn in teams – introducing interprofessional learning at the University Medical Centre Mannheim, Germany. GMS J Med Educ 33. https://doi.org/10.3205/zma001030

Quintero GA (2014) Medical education and the healthcare system – why does the curriculum need to be reformed? BMC Med 12. https://doi.org/10.1186/s12916-014-0213-3

Sergiovanni TJ (1996) Leadership for the schoolhouse: how is it different? why is it important? Wiley, San Francisco

Sherrin J (2000) A literature review exploring a meaning for the term "curriculum leadership". Waikato J Educ 6:133–141

Supe A, Burdick WP (2006) Challenges and issues in medical education in India. Acad Med J Assoc Am Med Coll 81:1076–1080. https://doi.org/10.1097/01.ACM.0000246699.94234.ab

Thompson KV, Chmielewski J, Gaines MS, Hrycyna CA, LaCourse WR (2013) Competency-based reforms of the undergraduate biology curriculum: integrating the physical and biological sciences. CBE Life Sci Educ 12:162–169. https://doi.org/10.1187/cbe.12-09-0143

Till A, McKimm J, Swanwick T (2017) Twelve tips for integrating leadership development into undergraduate medical education. Med Teach:1–7. https://doi.org/10.1080/0142159X.2017.1392009

10 Curriculum Committee

Objectives
1. To understand the need for central governance of undergraduate medical curriculum.
2. To describe the organizational structure of a curriculum committee.
3. To appreciate the functions of curriculum committee.

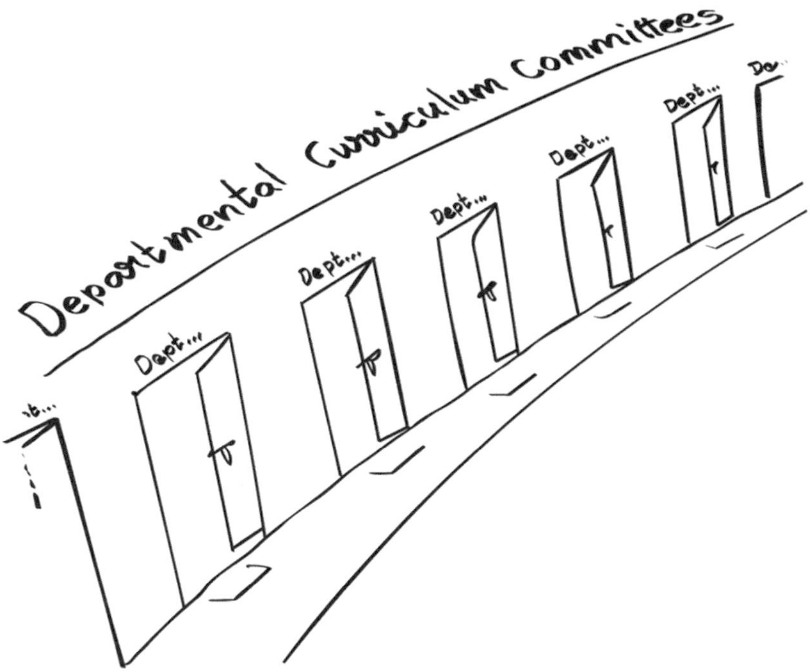

Fig. 10.1 Curriculum committee–as it is

Kadambari D et al., *Improving Discipline-Based Undergraduate Medical Curriculum*, https://doi.org/10.1007/978-981-13-1310-3_10

10.1 Introduction

A medical curriculum is a plan of educational experiences offered to a learner under the guidance of a recognized medical school. Curriculum is the blueprint for what students need to know and be able to do. It is the curriculum that sets the standards and requirements to fulfil those standards to achieve excellence in medical education. All medical schools must demonstrate leadership of medical education and training through effective educational governance (Casiro and Regehr 2017). 'Educational governance is the systems and standards through which organisations control their educational activities and demonstrate accountability for and the continuous improvement of the quality of education' (Solarsh et al. 2012).

Educational governance may be part of a wider, integrated governance framework comprising elements such as educational audit, clinical audit and organizational development. Coward (2010) says that the more integrated these elements are within the overall governance of the organization, the more effective educational governance is.

There are several domains of the educational governance such as the planning committee, budgeting committee and the curriculum committee out of which the curriculum committee is one of the major domains. The responsibility of the curriculum committee is to define the goals and objectives of the curriculum, for the design, management and evaluation of the undergraduate medical curriculum with respect to the mission and vision of the medical school and also in accordance with the accreditation requirements if any. Bertoncello et al. (2015) define the role of the curriculum as the integration of educational, clinical and medical governance to keep patients and learners safe and create an appropriate learning environment and organizational culture.

To ensure that the curriculum is coherent, coordinated, current and effective, it is the responsibility of the curriculum committee to establish the process of reviewing, evaluating and revising the curriculum on a recurring timeline. The other additional responsibility of the committee is to make recommendations to the dean about the system of incentives for teaching effort, support for teaching, research and extension work of faculty, teaching space required by the curriculum design and other support requirements needed to make the curriculum operational. With the approval of the dean, the committee has the authority of setting educational objectives, establishing educational requirements, allocating curriculum time, specifying teaching methods, selecting course coordinators or directors and evaluating educational outcomes. Carter et al. (2011) and Steyer et al. (2003) say that in addition to all this, the authority of setting performance standards for faculty, initiating faculty development efforts and evaluating faculty performance lies with the curriculum committee.

10.2 Need for Central Governance of Undergraduate Medical Curriculum

The traditional approach of departmental governance does not accommodate a broad integrative view of general undergraduate medical education due to the absence of mechanisms for horizontal and vertical integration (Reynolds et al. 1995).

The various academic disciplines tend not to identify strongly with the broader educational mission of the school and thus may not have a clear sense of specific goals and objectives appropriate for the undergraduate medical student. The departmental governance tends to be more educationally conservative, perhaps because it tends to reinforce departmental identity and generate resistance to cross-disciplinary and novel approaches. The departmental governance lacks broad peer review and accountability. In contrary, central governance of curriculum allows the introduction of new initiatives in a coordinated and timely fashion and provides a mechanism for dealing with the issues in curriculum. Central governance of curriculum facilitates systematic quality control, increased ability to identify areas of overlap and opportunities to foster longitudinal integration, ability to revise and take corrective action quickly, based on considerations of mission, ability to assign faculty responsibilities more fairly, evaluation of students and faculty input, programme evaluation, and establish a mechanism for creating a budget for general medical education (Bertoncello et al. 2015; Coward 2010; Reynolds et al. 1995).

10.3 Structure of Curriculum Governance

The general policy of the curriculum committee should be that it will oversee the entire educational programme leading to MBBS degree. The overall design, implementation, management and evaluation of a coherent and coordinated curriculum will be the responsibility of the curriculum committee. The dean who is the academic head of the institution will be chairperson of the curriculum governance committee. The curriculum governance committee shall consist of subcommittees interrelated to each other to provide oversight and governance of the medical school curriculum. These subcommittees may be named as the executive curriculum committee (ECC), foundational course curriculum committee (FCCC), basic sciences curriculum committee (BSCC), clinical sciences curriculum committee (CSCC) and curriculum evaluation committee (CEC). The foundational course curriculum committee, basic sciences curriculum committee, clinical sciences curriculum committee and curriculum evaluation committee will report to the executive curriculum committee, and the executive curriculum committee will report to the dean. All the subcommittees will support the mission of other committees (Al Shawwa 2012; Carter et al. 2011; Silkens et al. 2017).

10.4 Membership to Curriculum Committee

The dean.

The registrar.

Department heads and/or senior professor of the department.

Faculty from the department of medical education or faculty and administrators dedicated to education and with expertise in curricular design, pedagogy and evaluation methods.

Departmental representatives from all disciplines.

Faculty members with interest or expertise in curriculum development and/or assessment and who have done special courses in medical education technologies.

Member from information and communication technology unit.

Student representatives elected by students and/or interns.

The tenure of the membership will be for a period of at least 3 years except for the student representatives who are selected on a yearly basis.

10.5 Functions of Curriculum Committee

The curriculum committees must assure that the curriculum as a whole will be designed to achieve the educational objectives of the MBBS programme. Evidence of a coherent and coordinate curriculum includes:

Logical sequencing of the various segments of the curriculum.

Content that is coordinated and integrated within and across the academic periods of study (horizontal and vertical integration).

Methods of pedagogy and student evaluation that are appropriate for the achievement of the educational objectives.

Hence, the activities of the curriculum are centred around the above things, and the responsibilities of the curriculum committee include leading, directing, coordinating, controlling, planning, evaluating and revising the curriculum and reporting to the dean.

The general functions of the curriculum committee shall be to:

- Advise the dean on all matters concerning undergraduate medical education.
- Set the strategic direction for the delivery and assessment of the undergraduate medical course and develop the teaching and learning plan.
- Plan, coordinate and oversee the administration of teaching, learning and assessment arrangements for undergraduates in medicine according to the teaching and learning plan.
- Manage the teaching budget.
- Quality assure the undergraduate programme to meet the curricular objectives.
- Address and implement any required changes arising from the curriculum reviews.
- Provide leadership in curriculum development at the medical college.
- Provide a forum for innovation in teaching and learning.
- Review programmes and courses in a systematic manner on a regular basis to ensure that they are kept current and relevant.

The charge of each of the subcommittees is detailed, as follows:

10.6 Executive Curriculum Committee

It is the role of the ECC to develop the curriculum, to implement new ideas and to evaluate the existing curriculum of the medical school.

It is also the responsibility of the ECC to provide oversight to all the committees that report to it such as the preclinical committee, paraclinical committee, clinical committee and Curriculum Evaluation Committee.

The components of a good ECC are the best horizontal and vertical organization, design and integration.

The periodic review of the vertically integrated programmes, including but not limited to clinical skills, patient safety, inter-professional education, ethics, professionalism and cultural competency, is an important responsibility of the ECC.

It is also essential that the ECC reviews the entire curriculum for the COM, periodically, i.e. at least annually.

In order to maintain the highest standard of education for all its programmes, the ECC must develop specific educational programmes objectives/core competencies and must also periodically review them.

The ECC is also responsible for aligning the educational programme objectives/core competencies with the stated mission of the medical school.

In institutions looking to enhance the quality of teaching and further the mission of the medical school, the ECC must identify specific resources needed by the faculty and the students.

Another responsibility of the ECC is to monitor the content and workload in every discipline including the identification of omissions and redundancies. It is the duty of the committee to make sure that the standards of content in every academic period remain common. Regardless of the subsequent career specialty, the depth and breadth of the knowledge required for a general professional education must be addressed by these standards.

In order to assess and analyse the quality of its educational programme, various curriculum-related outcomes data must be periodically reviewed by the ECC.

Committees functioning under the ECC must hand over periodic reports and recommendations, if an, to the ECC. The recommendations put forth by the committees must be considered for discussion by the members of the ECC, and relevant issues must be submitted to the dean within the time limit of 60 days, for the welfare of the committees.

The reports submitted to the dean on the meetings held by the committee must contain information about the committee's activities, findings and recommendations.

10.7 Basic Sciences Curriculum Committee

It is the responsibility of the basic sciences curriculum committee to align the course with specific educational programme objectives/core competencies of the medical school.

It is the responsibility of the basic sciences curriculum committee to review the stated objectives of the individual educational experiences in each course as well as methods of pedagogy and student assessment, to assure congruence with educational programme objectives/core competencies of the institution.

The basic sciences curriculum committee must periodically review its course content, the educational course objectives and evaluations and consider changes in the curriculum based on feedback from students and faculty.

The basic sciences curriculum committee will include systems codirectors and thread directors as well as faculty with interest and expertise in the delivery of the relevant curriculum.

10.8 Clinical Sciences Curriculum Committee

It is the responsibility of the clinical sciences curriculum committee to align the clinical clerkships with specific educational programme objectives of the medical school.

It is the responsibility of the clinical sciences curriculum committee to review the stated objectives of the individual educational experiences in each clerkship as well as methods of pedagogy and student evaluation, to assure congruence with educational programme objectives of this institution.

The clinical sciences curriculum committee must develop, implement and monitor policies related to the amount of time students spend in required activities, including the total required hours spent in clinical and educational activities during clinical clerkships.

The clinical sciences curriculum committee must review guidelines regarding the requirements for adequacy of clinical experiences in each required clerkship and comparisons across clerkship sites.

The clinical sciences curriculum committee must monitor the student performance in years 3 and 4 related to medical knowledge, clinical skills and professionalism. Institutional and national benchmarks should be used for comparative analysis (Carter et al. 2011; Kako and Rudge 2008; Steyer et al. 2003).

10.9 Curriculum Evaluation Committee

It is the responsibility of the curriculum evaluation committee to periodically at regular intervals of not more than a year evaluate the curriculum and recommend changes to the executive curriculum committee based on these evaluations.

The curriculum evaluation committee must evaluate effectiveness of programmes by outcome analysis, using national norms of accomplishments as a frame of reference, supplemented by other objective and subjective methods of evaluation.

The responsibility of this committee is to evaluate courses and internship (clerkships in the curriculum, measured against: student feedback, end of course student performance, passing the qualifying examination for higher education, etc. All courses and internships are evaluated annually for the courses and educator quality (Kaufman 1998).

The curriculum evaluation committee must monitor the performance and content of the curriculum by reviewing an annual report submitted by each system by the beginning of the academic year. Recommendations based on evaluation of these annual reports should be submitted to the relevant curriculum committee within 90 days of receipt of such (Kako and Rudge 2008; Reynolds et al. 1995; Wilkes and Bligh 1999).

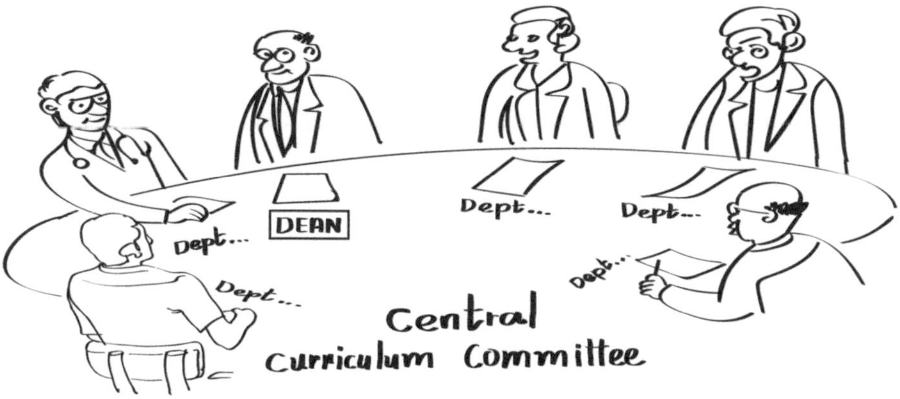

Fig. 10.2 Curriculum committee–as it should be

Conclusion

It is the responsibility of a well-governed curriculum to help an institution assess the effectiveness of the curriculum at regular intervals. The curriculum committee is responsible for defining the goals and objectives of the curriculum, for the design, management and evaluation of the undergraduate medical curriculum in accordance with the mission and vision of the medical school and also in accordance with the accreditation requirements if any. Until the curriculum committee documents the various activities conducted by it, the reformation or the introduction of any change in the existing curriculum will not be a difficult task. In order to keep patients and learners safe and create an appropriate learning environment and organizational culture, it is essential for the curriculum committee to work with the other committees, leading to the integration of educational, clinical and medical governance. It is the responsibility of the curriculum committee to review, evaluate and revise the curriculum at regular intervals to make sure that the curriculum is current, coherent, coordinated and effective.

References

Al Shawwa LA (2012) The establishment and roles of the Medical Education Department in the Faculty of Medicine, King Abdul Aziz University, Jeddah Saudi Arabia. Oman Med J 27:4–9. https://doi.org/10.5001/omj.2012.02

Bertoncello C, Buja A, Silenzi A, Specchia ML, Franchino G, Lazzari A, Baldo V, Ricciardi W, Damiani G (2015) Good governance competencies in public health to train public health physicians. Int J Public Health 60:737–749. https://doi.org/10.1007/s00038-015-0702-y

Carter JT, Draugalis JR, Bruce SP, Gonyeau MR (2011) The role of curriculum committees in pharmacy education. Am J Pharm Educ 75. https://doi.org/10.5688/ajpe758154

Casiro O, Regehr G (2017) Enacting pedagogy in curricula: on the vital role of governance in medical education. Acad Med J Assoc Am Med Coll. https://doi.org/10.1097/ACM.0000000000001774

Coward R (2010) Educational governance in the NHS: a literature review. Int J Health Care Qual Assur 23:708–717. https://doi.org/10.1108/09526861011081840

Kako M, Rudge T (2008) Governing nursing: curriculum as a rhetorical vehicle using South Australian nursing schools from the 1950s onwards as an illustrative case. Contemp Nurse 30:142–155

Kaufman A (1998) Leadership and governance. Acad Med 73:S11

Reynolds CF, Adler S, Kanter SL, Horn JP, Harvey J, Bernier GM (1995) The undergraduate medical curriculum: centralized versus departmentalized. Acad Med J Assoc Am Med Coll 70:671–675

Silkens MEWM, Lombarts KMJMH, Scherpbier AJJA, Heineman MJ, Arah OA (2017) Towards healthy learning climates in postgraduate medical education: exploring the role of hospital-wide education committees. BMC Med Educ 17:241. https://doi.org/10.1186/s12909-017-1075-0

Solarsh G, Lindley J, Whyte G, Fahey M, Walker A (2012) Governance and assessment in a widely distributed medical education program in Australia. Acad Med J Assoc Am Med Coll 87:807–814. https://doi.org/10.1097/ACM.0b013e318253226a

Steyer TE, Ravenell RL, Mainous AG, Blue AV (2003) The role of medical students in curriculum committees. Teach Learn Med 15:238–241. https://doi.org/10.1207/S15328015TLM1504_04

Wilkes M, Bligh J (1999) Evaluating educational interventions. BMJ 318:1269–1272

Faculty Development

11

Objectives
1. To understand the expanding roles of medical teachers.
2. To explain the role of faculty development programmes for developing better teachers.
3. To list the steps in designing a faculty development programme.
4. To identify content/topics for faculty development that emphasizes teaching, learning and assessment.
5. To suggest a framework for organizing faculty development programmes.

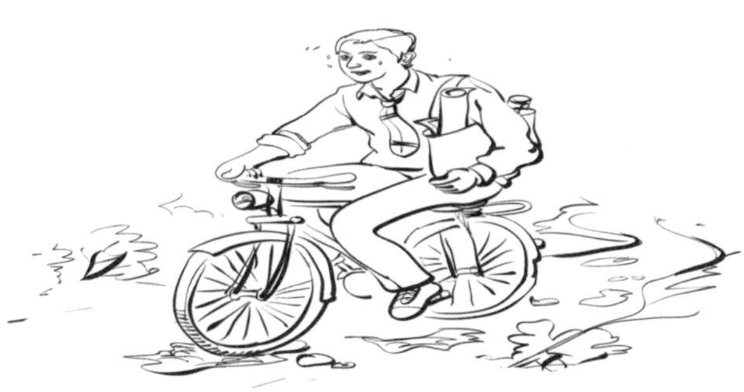

Fig. 11.1 Before faculty development

"Burdensome preparation and transaction of content"

Kadambari D et al., *Improving Discipline-Based Undergraduate Medical Curriculum*, https://doi.org/10.1007/978-981-13-1310-3_11

11.1 Introduction

Faculty development is an organized, goal-directed process to achieve career progression and growth. Inherent in this process is the acquisition of skills that enable one to contribute in a meaningful way to the advancement of a field of interest, whether educational, operational or scientific. The process requires attention to technical skills, personal attributes and explicit goals. Supportive mentorship is optimal (Hamilton and Brown 2003).

The most essential element in the effectiveness of an institution in higher education is faculty development. Faculty development plays a prominent role at many medical institutions across the globe. Faculty development can be broadly defined as any activity that contributes to the skills of faculty members or aids in their professional advancement. According to Hamilton and Brown (2003) and Walling (1999), faculty development may also include a wide array of activities. Improving teaching skills, fostering research and facilitating professional advancement are various factors focused upon by the most traditional faculty development programs. Amin et al. (2009) believe that these kinds of traditional faculty development programs are often centred at academic institutions based on an institutional level where faculty members belonging to various sectors of the institution are trained according to their professional requirements.

As far as medical education is concerned, the level of student engagement, motivation and learning will be strongly influenced by the support of the medical college to its faculty development. The faculty members who strive towards professional development will get to experience increased vitality, informed pedagogy, teaching innovations and scholarly teaching. Moreover, faculty professional development contributes to the effective use of emerging technologies and establishes a firm foundation for the overall development of high-quality programs and curricula. In today's education system with its rapidly changing knowledge base, the fast advancing technologies and the unique characteristics of today's learners, it is all demanded of the medical teachers that they give high priority to their own professional development. Amin et al. (2009) and Skeff et al. (1997) say that a university's finding of effective ways to motivate and reward faculty participation is also demanded by the technological developments and characteristics of today's learners.

Medical education reform is a continuous process in response to advances in medical care and increased demands from patients and the medical environment. The prominent aim of the MBBS programs offered in the current situation is to promote competency in general practice skills in the new generation of physicians with a holistic perspective of patient-centred medicine. This has led to the adaptation of new methodologies in medical schools in the admission process, curricular design, educational strategies and assessment. However, the teaching-learning scenario remains the same as it was before a few decades, even though the quantum of knowledge has increased manyfold and the emergence of newer technologies in teaching and learning are rapidly proliferating. Therefore, Al Shawwa (2012) and Steinert et al. (2012) put forth the idea that in order to promote learning and application of the core competencies established by the apex medical education implementation bodies, it is essential to organize faculty development program in all medical institutions.

The aim of the faculty development program is to empower the competencies of faculties in teaching the core competences proposed by the apex bodies of medical education. The ultimate goal of faculty development is to promote change in individuals, curriculum and institutions. At the individual level, a good faculty development program facilitates knowledge acquisition, attitudinal change and skill development in medical education (Skeff et al. 1997). For those who already excel in teaching, the program can enhance the quality of teaching and introduce new effective teaching behaviours and concepts of medical education. At the curriculum development level, teachers trained in small groups are more prone to modify teaching behaviour while providing a variety of teaching skills or attitude. At the institution level, the faculty development program brings change to the teaching atmosphere and leads to quality improvement in the whole organization (Steinert et al. 2012).

Medical education has seen major changes over the past decade. Integrated teaching, problem-based learning, community-based learning, core curriculum with electives and systematic curriculum planning have been advocated (Davis et al. 2017). Students are expected to take more responsibility for their learning and more emphasis is given for self-directed learning. Technological advancements have brought in a paradigm shift in the delivery of medical education, and new directions in the assessment of students 'for learning' and 'of learning' with more emphasis on performance assessment have compelled the medical teachers to play different types of roles for achieving the stated goals of medical education (Davis et al. 2005).

The different roles a medical teacher is expected to play are:

1. Provider of information—teacher or a facilitator in a practical or clinical setting, lecturer in a classroom setting.
2. Role model—on-the-job role model, role model as a professor.
3. Facilitator—mentor, personal advisor or tutor providing assistance to students in learning.
4. Examiner or assessor—one who plans formal examinations for the students and also evaluates the curriculum.
5. Developer of resources—develops resource materials for study guides, making it easier for the students to learn by themselves from the computer or from the soft copy of the guides or resources.
6. Planner—one who organizes the course and plans the curriculum.

The management of multiple roles and new responsibilities like clinical instruction, micro group teaching and problem-based tutorials and case-based discussions falls upon the faculty members of the modern-day medical colleges. It is also the responsibility of the faculty members to become mentors and develop and evaluate new curricula, to integrate technology into teaching and to learn and research and master new computer-based educational programs. Al Shawwa (2012) and Bakhshialiabad et al. (2015) feel that the faculty should also demonstrate leadership and management proficiency. Therefore, faculty development programs should be organized in every institution for the faculty members in order to prepare them to deal with the rapid changes and shifting paradigms in medical education, healthcare delivery systems and clinical practice. Lack of such training will make teachers look like mere instructors presenting their understanding of the subject through one-way lectures.

The main goals of faculty development programs are to teach the faculty members the skills relevant to their institutional setting and their position of faculty and to sustain their vitality both now and in the future (Elzubeir 2011).

Adkoli and Sood (2009), Skeff et al. (1997), and Walling (1999) state that the three main factors which make a faculty development programme successful are the determination of the measurement of success of the FDP, the identification of the area(s) for faculty development and the identification of the target audience(s).

11.2 Steps in Designing a Faculty Development Programme

Understand the institutional/organizational culture.
Determine appropriate goals and priorities.
Conduct needs assessments to ensure relevant programming.
Develop different programs to accommodate diverse needs.
Incorporate principles of adult learning and instructional design.
Offer a diversity of educational methods.
Work to overcome commonly encountered challenges.
Prepare resource faculty.
Evaluate and demonstrate effectiveness of the programme.

11.3 Content for Faculty Development that Emphasizes Teaching, Learning and Assessment

Syllabus and course design.
Writing objectives.
Constructing assessments.
Rubric designing.
Grading strategies.
Student motivation.
Learning disabilities.
Classroom management.
Active learning methods.
Presentation and communication skills.
Self-reflection.
Searching and evaluating evidence.
Scholarship in teaching.
Educational leadership.
Educational research.

11.4 Format of Faculty Development Programmes

(1) Organizational strategies, (2) fellowships, (3) comprehensive local programmes, (4) workshops and seminars, (5) continuing medical education and (6) individual activities.

Workshops.
Short-term courses.
Long-term courses.

Fellowship courses.
Online self-directed learning.

11.5 Common Challenges

Defining goals and priorities.
Balancing individual needs and organizational needs.
Motivating faculty to join the faculty development programmes.
Training the resource faculty.
Working within limited resources.
Choosing appropriate methods and formats for the workshop.
Sustaining the relevancy and practical delivery of the programme.
Obtaining institutional and other stakeholders support.

11.6 Areas for Assessing the Effectiveness of Faculty Development Programme

The impact of a faculty development program should be measured by a thorough and focused assessment plan in terms of:

Overall satisfaction of the participants and other stakeholders.
Desirable changes in attitudes towards teaching and other faculty development noted.
Acquired knowledge, attitude and skills.
Changes in teaching and teacher behaviours as reported and observed.
Changes in student learning and organizational practice as reported and observed.
Ability in utilizing the learning opportunities within and outside the institution.
Ability to mobilize teaching-learning resources and create teaching-learning resources.
Adopt and adapt to innovative educational practices.
Appraising the quality of educational activities.
Undertake educational leadership roles.

11.7 Future Directions

Future faculty development programmes should aim at moving beyond the improvement of teaching/instructional and assessment improvement by focusing on developing alternate 'models' of faculty development using technological inputs. Importance should also be given to framing theoretical framework for faculty development in all respects. Contemporary organizational climate should be taken into consideration to promote faculty development through collaborative education and online education. Finally evaluating the effectiveness of faculty development programme using robust and vibrant methods will help the faculty development organizations to take the faculty development programmes forward in all respects.

Fig. 11.2 After faculty development

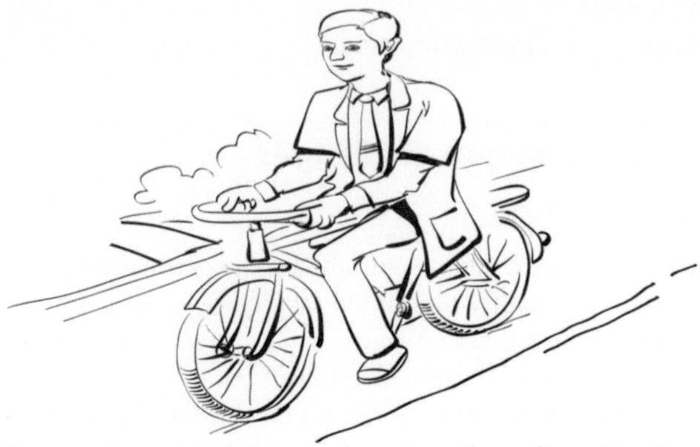

Conclusion

Faculty teaching development programmes are beneficial as has been measured through surveys and student evaluations. Programmes increase faculty members' value of teaching, rekindle their motivation and enthusiasm and improve their knowledge, behaviours and dissemination of skills. Faculty development programmes that support teaching improvement, effectiveness and competency are needed for individuals teaching in colleges and schools of pharmacy because excellent teachers are needed in order to prepare future pharmacists to advance the practice and become essential members of the healthcare team who practice at the top of their license. Several faculty development models can be implemented to support teaching development, and there is evidence that faculty development in this arena is effective. After a careful analysis of the benefits and costs associated with the models, faculty members can make informed decisions about which faculty teaching development plan would be most appropriately and successfully implemented at their institution. More research is necessary to maximize the outcomes of faculty development programs.

References

Adkoli BV, Sood R (2009) Faculty development and medical education units in India: a survey. Natl Med J India 22:28–32

Al Shawwa LA (2012) The establishment and roles of the Medical Education Department in the Faculty of Medicine, King Abdul Aziz University, Jeddah Saudi Arabia. Oman Med J 27:4–9. https://doi.org/10.5001/omj.2012.02

Amin Z, Eng KH, Seng CY, Hoon TC, Sun GP, Samarasekera DD, Huak CY, Rhoon KD (2009) A multi-institutional survey on faculty development needs, priorities and preferences in medical education in an Asian medical school. Med Educ Online 14:16. https://doi.org/10.3885/meo.2009.Res00317

Bakhshialiabad H, Bakhshi M, Hassanshahi G (2015) Students' perceptions of the academic learning environment in seven medical sciences courses based on DREEM. Adv Med Educ Pract 6:195–203. https://doi.org/10.2147/AMEP.S60570

Davis MH, Karunathilake I, Harden RM (2005) AMEE Education Guide no. 28: the development and role of departments of medical education. Med Teach 27:665–675. https://doi.org/10.1080/01421590500398788

Davis BW, Gooden MA, Bowers AJ (2017) Pathways to the principalship: an event history analysis of the careers of teachers with principal certification. Am Educ Res J 54:207–240. https://doi.org/10.3102/0002831216687530

Elzubeir M (2011) Faculty-led faculty development: evaluation and reflections on a distributed educational leadership model. Saudi J Kidney Dis Transplant 22:90–96

Hamilton GC, Brown JE (2003) Faculty development: what is faculty development? Acad Emerg Med 10:1334–1336

Skeff KM, Stratos GA, Mygdal W, DeWitt TA, Manfred L, Quirk M, Roberts K, Greenberg L, Bland CJ (1997) Faculty development. J Gen Intern Med 12:S56–S63. https://doi.org/10.1046/j.1525-1497.12.s2.8.x

Steinert Y, Naismith L, Mann K (2012) Faculty development initiatives designed to promote leadership in medical education. A BEME systematic review: BEME Guide No. 19. Med Teach 34:483–503. https://doi.org/10.3109/0142159X.2012.680937

Walling AD (1999) Medical education 101—a faculty development course. Acad Med J Assoc Am Med Coll 74:609

Student Support

12

Objectives

1. To state the nature of student support services.
2. To stress the need for student support services.
3. To explain the different domains of student support services.

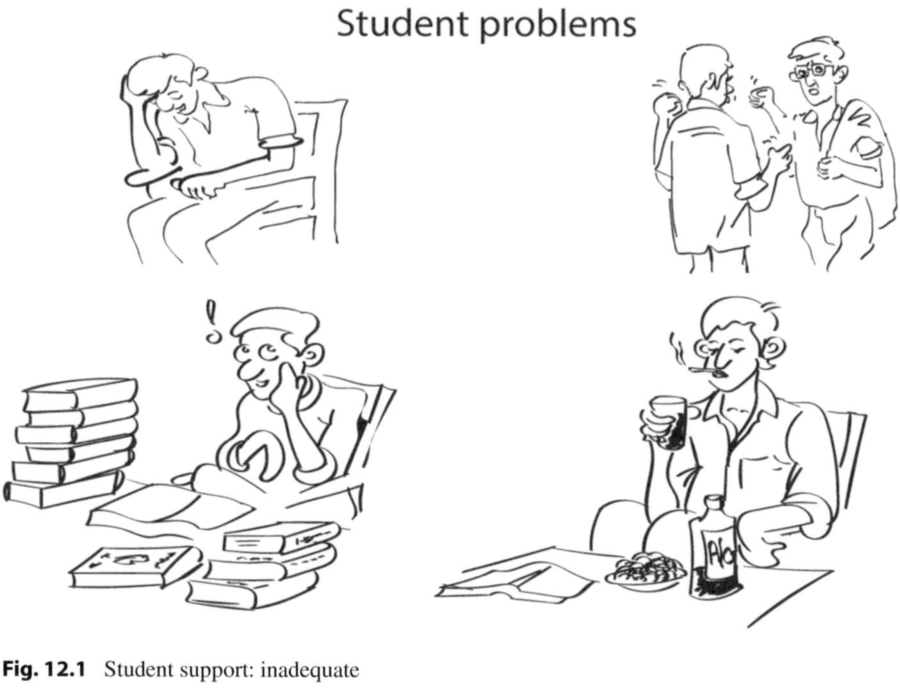

Fig. 12.1 Student support: inadequate

Kadambari D et al., *Improving Discipline-Based Undergraduate Medical Curriculum*, https://doi.org/10.1007/978-981-13-1310-3_12

12.1 Introduction

Being a student of a medical college is different from being a student of other disciplines or other professional colleges for a medical college has its own characteristics that differentiates the learning experience and learning environment of other institutions of higher learning. Here the needs of the students are different, and it demands a wide variety of approaches and services to develop them as a medical professional (Hays et al. 2011; Vogan et al. 2014). Academically bright and ambitious medical students must cope with a combination of curriculum, assessment, career choice, personal, family and social pressures. Many seek support, and some present complex problems that consume substantial resources. A few continue unresolved into postgraduate life and may affect future professional performance (Vogan et al. 2014). We want our students to succeed in the classroom, in the clinics and in life. Medical students often require high levels of specialized institutional and personal support to facilitate success. Contributory factors may include personality type, course pressures and financial hardship. Early intervention in the form of student support services may be helpful in minimising the impact on both individual students and school resources. The very purpose of these support services is to make the students feel that they are not alone or helpless during the period of their study. They should be made to feel that they are a member of a well organized institution which is ready to help them whenever they need help in order to complete their professional degree successfully (Hays et al. 2011). This section will review how a medical college can provide the required support services effectively.

12.2 Academic Support Services

Academic environment—faculty should be well prepared to provide academic support on reading, writing, identifying learning resources, effective use of leaning resources, self-assessment, further learning, etc. among their students. Academic counsellors can identify and recommend effective learning environments that are conducive for their students learning (Bakhshialiabad et al. 2015; Casiro and Regehr 2017).

Academic counselling—appointment of academic counsellor and mentors will help the institution to achieve the goals of academic support services. The academic counsellors and mentors should be provided with relevant training in these areas that will enable them to do justice for their position (Ciobanu 2013; Vogan et al. 2014).

Learning circles—formation of student academic support network will also make the academic support services more visible and enhance participation of more members. Learning circles are a highly interactive, participatory structure for organizing group work. The goal is to build, share and express knowledge through a process of open dialogue and deep reflection around issues or problems with a focus on a shared outcome. Online learning circles are teams of distance learners who use technology to acquire a deeper understanding of areas of shared interest. The structure balances individual ownership with collective responsibility to provide a setting which helps everyone achieve their learning objectives. The circle is managed by distributed leadership and suggests that each participant be engaged in leading one of the group projects. They can be used in a wide range of formal and informal contexts (Learning Circle Model—Online Learning Circles, nd). Peer mentors can be trained to provide academic guidance to their peers.

12.3 Library Services

Medical students should have 24 × 7 ready access to library services and library resources. For this a well maintained library with all print and electronic resources with latest learning technology and electronic learning environment to support the educational goals of the students should be in place. The library should also serve as a centre that fosters appropriate learning with resources more focussed on learners current learning needs (Sherwill-Navarro and Wallace 2004).

12.4 Information Technology Resources and Services

Information technology has become part and parcel of everyone's life, and the present generation students are tech-savvy and are well informed in applying technology in their day-to-day activities. Al-Tamimi (2003) believes that, in order to provide the learners the access to information and in order to help them communicate their needs from anywhere and at anytime, it is the responsibility of the medical colleges to provide them with updated communication technology resources and to provide them up-to-date information on the subjects. These services may include mass media education, using portable electronic gadgets effectively for learning, e-learning, m-learning, virtual learning environments, etc.; the maintenance of portfolio, the formative examinations and a part or the whole of summative examinations can be made computer based. Houshyari et al. (2012a, b) say that the availability of classroom lectures and activities online through the institute intranet services is also essential to facilitate learning from anywhere and at anytime.

12.5 Learning Spaces

Appropriate designing of classroom spaces and other learning spaces such as study lounge at college and at hostel, sit-outs in the lawn and walking paths can be arranged to facilitate the mood for learning. The learning spaces should be made in such a way that it should be conducive for learning through group discussions and other group activities (Bakhshialiabad et al. 2015).

12.6 Service Learning

Medical students should be prepared for their role as healthcare providers, community leaders, collaborators, mentors and educators in the community they work. Service learning is a method of experiential learning. Medical students meet community health needs while developing their own ability to understand and address the complex health challenges they will encounter in patient care. The medical college should ensure that the medical education programme provides sufficient opportunities that encourage and support medical student participation in service learning and community service activities. Specific programmes to motivate students to participate in socially relevant and useful programmes that promote service learning should be in place. Medical colleges should develop a framework for inculcating service learning among their learners. This includes identifying community partners, service learning projects and service learning environments (Ciobanu 2013; Hays et al. 2011; Kollhoff et al. 2015).

12.7 Research Support Services

A contemporary medical curriculum is conducted in an environment that fosters intellectual challenge and spirit of inquiry in the field of medicine and allied health sciences. Sufficient opportunities, encouragement and support for medical students participation in research and other scholarly activities should be taken care by setting a division for research exclusively for budding scholars. This division will take care of sensitizing and training the students to take part in basic sciences and clinical research conducted in the institute and its partner institutions and foster scientific temper. The research division will also be responsible for conducting orientation programme in research methodology, summer/winter training programmes, poster presentation, journal article presentation, conference presentations and other activities that promotes scientific temper among the students (Huhn et al. 2015).

12.8 Services for Medical Personality Development and Development of Soft Skills

Medical personality is a dynamic and organized set of characteristics that uniquely influence the society which are to be developed among the medical students. These traits play an important role as the doctor-patient relation is unique and sacred and bound by emotions of society. Therefore, the medical institution has to play a key role by exposing students to the community that will provide teaching and learning opportunities for the development of soft skills. Soft skills include professional, interpersonal and social skills, communication skills and professional and ethical attitudes. A well-planned communication and personality development programme to update the students for the highly competitive future should be offered by the medical colleges (Sandars et al. 2014).

12.9 Student Safety, Security and Disaster Preparedness

Safety and security should be the high priority in any medical college, and unless these security needs are fulfilled adequately, the students will not show interest in their learning. Every medical college should have adequate security systems located at various places in the campus and must publish policies and procedures to ensure student safety. These colleges must also be prepared for emergency situations and must effectively address issues regarding exposure to infectious and environmental hazards through pre-planned policies and guidelines. Humphrey (2010) and Paul et al. (2009) insist that in order to enhance the safety and security of the students in a medical institution, security personnel should be deployed in clinics, workplace, parking and other student movement areas and emergency phones should also be installed in these areas. They also feel that the phone numbers of quick response team must be made aware to all and that the institutions must have proper fire safety equipments installed.

12.10 Personal and Career Guidance and Counselling Services

Guidance and counselling services should be available to provide guidance and counselling on the personal and career issues of the students. Counsellors will provide assistance and guidance to students in order to help them achieve personal and academic success. Stecker (2004) and Yiu (2005) list out the various benefits of counselling. They say that counselling helps in the evaluation of academic performance, provides sources for financial assistance, helps improve relationships with friends and family and contributes to the overall well-being of the student by helping him/her manage stress better. All concerns of the students must be taken seriously, and there should be such a mechanism that all their voices are heard, questions are answered and problems are solved. An effective career advising system should be in place that integrates the efforts of faculty members to assist medical students in choosing elective courses, evaluating career options and applying to residency programmes. Periodic programmes to promote student well-being and to facilitate their adjustment to the physical and emotional demands of medical education should also be a part of the guidance and counselling services.

12.11 Student Healthcare Services

Medical students' well-being is an essential part of their educational success. Timely access to needed diagnostic, preventative and therapeutic health services at sites in reasonable proximity to their locations should be in place. The medical college should have necessary arrangements in place to provide primary care as well as urgent care services to their students. Immunization guidelines and guidelines for health insurance should be given to all the students as part of preventive health services and to promote their well-being (Yiu 2005).

Fig. 12.2 Student support: optimal

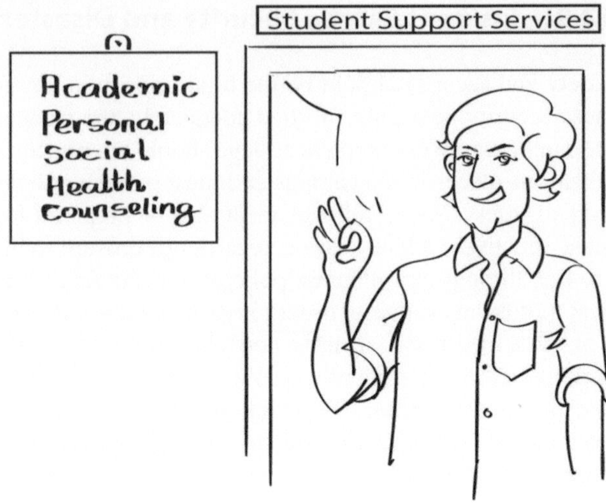

Conclusion

It is highly important that all the students in a medical college receive excellent medical education. Every medical institution should create an environment that fosters the educational process and provides the students with essential support services for a student's academic success may be directly correlated with how well the institution addresses student support services. In developing a medical college, considerable attention must be directed towards developing and implementing a curriculum, recruiting faculty and staff and constructing adequate medical education facilities.

References

Al-Tamimi DM (2003) Application of information and communication technologies in medical education. J Family Community Med 10:67–76

Bakhshialiabad H, Bakhshi M, Hassanshahi G (2015) Students' perceptions of the academic learning environment in seven medical sciences courses based on DREEM. Adv Med Educ Pract 6:195–203. https://doi.org/10.2147/AMEP.S60570

Casiro O, Regehr G (2017) Enacting pedagogy in curricula: on the vital role of governance in medical education. Acad Med J Assoc Am Med Coll. https://doi.org/10.1097/ACM.0000000000001774

Ciobanu A (2013) The role of student services in the improving of student experience in higher education. Procedia – Soc Behav Sci, Logos Universality Mentality Education Novelty (LUMEN 2013), Iasi, Romania, 10–13 Apr 2013 92, pp 169–173. https://doi.org/10.1016/j.sbspro.2013.08.654

Hays RB, Lawson M, Gray C (2011) Problems presented by medical students seeking support: a possible intervention framework. Med Teach 33:161–164. https://doi.org/10.3109/0142159X.2010.509415

Houshyari AB, Bahadorani M, Tootoonchi M, Gardiner JJZ, Peña RA, Adibi P (2012a) Medical education and information and communication technology. J Educ Health Promot 1. https://doi.org/10.4103/2277-9531.94411

Houshyari AB, Bahadorani M, Tootoonchi M, Gardiner JJZ, Peña RA, Adibi P (2012b) Information and communication technology in medical education: an experience from a developing country. JPMA J Pak Med Assoc 62:S71–S75

Huhn D, Junne F, Zipfel S, Duelli R, Resch F, Herzog W, Nikendei C (2015) International medical students – a survey of perceived challenges and established support services at medical faculties. GMS Z Für Med Ausbild 32. https://doi.org/10.3205/zma000951

Humphrey HJ (2010) Resources for medical education: finding the right prescription. Trans Am Clin Climatol Assoc 121:76–90 discussion 90–93

Kollhoff L, Kollhoff M, Cathcart-Rake W (2015) Providing support services for medical students on a rural regional medical campus. Med Sci Educ 25:157–162. https://doi.org/10.1007/s40670-015-0108-8

Learning Circle Model–Online Learning Circles [WWW Document] (n.d.) URL: https://sites.google.com/site/onlinelearningcircles/Home/learning-circles-defined. Accessed 3 Feb 2018

Paul G, Hinman G, Dottl S, Passon J (2009) Academic development: a survey of academic difficulties experienced by medical students and support services provided. Teach Learn Med 21:254–260. https://doi.org/10.1080/10401330903021041

Sandars J, Patel R, Steele H, McAreavey M, Association for Medical Education Europe (2014) Developmental student support in undergraduate medical education: AMEE Guide No. 92. Med Teach 36:1015–1026. https://doi.org/10.3109/0142159X.2014.917166

Sherwill-Navarro PJ, Wallace AL (2004) Research on the value of medical library services: does it make an impact in the health care literature? J Med Libr Assoc 92:34–42

Stecker T (2004) Well-being in an academic environment. Med Educ 38:465–478. https://doi.org/10.1046/j.1365-2929.2004.01812.x

Vogan CL, McKimm J, Da Silva AL, Grant A (2014) Twelve tips for providing effective student support in undergraduate medical education. Med Teach 36:480–485. https://doi.org/10.3109/0142159X.2014.907488

Yiu V (2005) Supporting the well-being of medical students. CMAJ Can Med Assoc J 172:889–890. https://doi.org/10.1503/cmaj.050126

13 Educational Environment

Objectives

1. Explain the meaning of 'learning environment'.
2. Forms of learning environments (formal, non-formal and informal).
3. Analyse different components of learning environment.
4. Understand various learning environments for all-round development of medical students.
5. Suggest guidelines to maintain and sustain a conducive learning environment in classrooms.

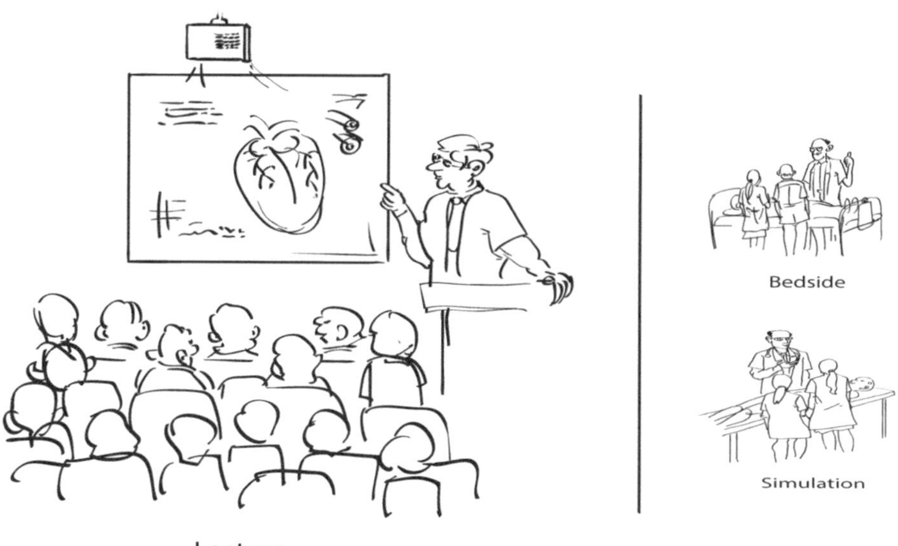

Fig. 13.1 Educational environment—as it is

Kadambari D et al., *Improving Discipline-Based Undergraduate Medical Curriculum*, https://doi.org/10.1007/978-981-13-1310-3_13

13.1 Introduction

Environment in which learning takes place may be described as a composite of natural conditions, circumstances and influences and sociocultural contexts in which an individual is situated. Therefore, we can say that learning environment is the sum total of the surroundings in which individuals interact to enrich experiences and thus leading to learning. Hutchinson (2003) says the most creative part of teaching is the development of a complete learning environment for students in a particular course or programme. Learning environment does not particularly have to mean the physical institutional learning environment or the personal learning environment. Spencer (2003) believes that a good learning environment has more to it than just these physical components. They will also include:

- The characteristics of the learners.
- The goals for teaching and learning.
- The activities that will best support learning.
- The assessment strategies that will best measure and drive learning.
- The culture that infuses the learning environment.

Medical schools should make sure that its medical education programme occurs in professional, respectful and intellectually stimulating academic and clinical environments. Wiskin et al. (2018) say that a medical institution should also make it a point to provide its students with the benefits of diversity in order to provide its students with the benefits of diversity in order for them to easily attain the qualities required by them to become future physicians. It is also important to understand that learning is not just an ongoing process which is only associated with schooling but is also a result of the interaction between individuals and the environments in which they operate.

Hence, it is a dynamic process, which takes place throughout life (Stewart 2006; Torre et al. 2006).

Environment in which learning takes place may be described as a composite of natural conditions, circumstances and influences and sociocultural contexts in which an individual is situated. Therefore, we can say that learning environment is the sum total of the surroundings in which individuals interact to enrich experiences and thus leading to learning (Remmen 1998).

13.2 'Learning Environment' from the Point of View of Various Learning Theories

Behaviourism concerns the observable change in behaviour. Behaviourists believe that learning is an explorative process which is provided by change in the actions or the behaviour of individuals. The process involves exposing the individuals to external stimuli until a desired response is received. Knowledge is usually transferred by the teacher, while the learner is a passive participant. Hartzell (2007) and Taylor and Hamdy (2013) consider knowledge to be objective, factual and absolute.

Cognitivism emerged when researchers found out that behaviourism did not account for all types of learning. According to the theory of cognitivism, knowledge can be viewed as the symbolic mental constructions that are organized or processed in the mind. Taylor and Hamdy (2013) believe that the learning process commences when the learner finally becomes an active participant.

Constructivism assumes that learning is a process of constructing knowledge rather than acquiring it. It takes the learner's social, cultural and contextual conditions into consideration and theorizes that the learner constructs knowledge through experience. Kaufman (2003) and Taylor and Hamdy (2013) say that according to this theory, learners assimilate new knowledge by reflecting on their contextual experiences which help them build on their existing knowledge.

Experiential learning theory is a holistic perspective on learning that combines experiences, perception, cognition and behaviour. The theory emphasizes the central role of experience in the learning process. According to Yardley et al. (2012), experiential learning theory is a continuous process grounded in experience.

Humanists have priority for human needs and interests. According to Colliver (2002) and Taylor and Hamdy (2013), humanists believe that as every individual grows and develops over the lifespan, it is necessary to study a person as a whole.

Social-situational theorists emphasize that learning takes place also in social relationships. Social learning theory posits that people learn from observing other people. By definition, such observations take place only in a social setting. Haddock (1994) says that according to Bandura, most human beings conceive ideas about new behaviours by observing other people's behaviours and use them as guidelines for their own actions.

If we analyse the various learning theories, we can find that social environment plays a significant role in learning. Bandura, a social psychologist, in his social learning theory proposed that new behaviour can be learnt through the process of observation and imitation. Therefore, it can be said that learning takes place as a result of interactions among personal characteristics, behaviour and environmental factors. Besides social environment, physical environment also influences learning. The role of culture is also considered as a significant factor of learning. Vygotsky, a constructivist thinker, believed that the mastery over the culturally important tasks can take place only through social interactions. For him, sociocultural environment plays a significant role in the process of learning as the learner uses cultural tools like language to mediate the meaning-making process. Thomas et al. (2014) say that variations in learning environment lead to different learning outcomes and that it is understood that the outcome of learning is contextual in nature.

Learning is a continuous process and is not limited to any particular setting. Based on the different types of settings, UNESCO (1984) classified the following types of learning:

- Formal learning—institutionalized.
- Non-formal learning—organized with flexibility.
- Informal learning—incidental and individualized, not organized.

13.2.1 Formal Learning Environment

Learning environment that occurs in formal organized institutions like schools, colleges and universities is known as formal learning environment. Formal learning institutions are highly structured in terms of learning objectives, learning time or learning support and aim at certification which leads to recognized qualification. The intention of learning process is very high from the perspective of the learner. The primary objective of formal education is to transmit the knowledge, skills, attitudes, beliefs, etc. preserved and propagated by a society. As a formal learning organization, medical school plays a major role in formation of ideas, habits and attitudes of a medical student with the aim of development of well-balanced professional personalities. The stakeholders in a medical school system include learners, parents, teachers, community and administration. Out of them teachers and students are two major stakeholders in a medical school system. The functioning of a medical school as a formal learning organization is characterized by the continuous interactions between students and teachers.

13.2.2 Informal Learning Environment

Learning environment which occurs in everyday life (at working place, in hospital, in the community, etc.) is called informal learning environment. Informal learning is not structured and does not aim at certification. In some cases, informal learning can occur with purposes, usually it is unintentional. There are many places that constitute informal environments of learning. Home is the first informal place of learning for a child. All of us know that a child learns a lot of life skills, attitudes, social manners and knowledge of his/her immediate world through his/her interaction with family members like mother, father, brothers, sisters and others. Informal learning enables children to change their behaviour from being self-centred to being socially aware, caring for the needs and rights of other family members. Gradually, the child is introduced to the social processes of the neighbourhood community of which the family is a part. Thus, the family, the neighbourhood community, the peer groups, the workplace, etc. form the informal learning environment that has profound impact on the sociocultural and cognitive development of the child. There are a number of factors which help in creating an appropriate learning environment at college; some of them are as follows:

- The number of books and other learning materials or resources at learning place.
- The amount of reward and recognition the students receive from their teachers for academic achievement.
- The teachers or parent's expectation regarding their students/wards academic achievement.
- An interactive learning environment where the stakeholders of medical education are able to provide facilitative learning environment for the learner helps the learner to grow cognitively and socially.

- Apart from home and college, community also plays an important role in providing informal learning environment to the learner.

13.2.3 Non-formal Learning Environment

Non-formal learning environment, unlike formal learning, takes place outside the formal educational structure. Non-formal learning intends to achieve predetermined educational objectives. But, unlike formal learning, non-formal learning always caters to the learning need of a specific target group. In a country, one can find a number of initiatives and programmes, which are non-formal by nature. In India, adult education programmes, basic education programmes, literacy programmes, health awareness programme, programmes meant for school dropouts, agricultural extension programmes and the like constitute non-formal learning programmes. Non-formal learning programmes are always conceptualized to achieve short-term and special educational goals and objectives. For example, in any kind of literacy programme, the objective is only to achieve literacy among the illiterates, and the programme is geared towards the achievement of that objective only. Curricular experiences in non-formal learning programmes are generally formulated keeping in mind the specific needs of the target group. These are more individualized rather than broad-based and general in nature. For example, programmes meant for village-level health workers contain specific information pertaining to healthcare in the context of village environment. The teaching-learning process is generally learner-oriented and flexible in nature. Transaction of learning experiences is centred around community resources. Activities in non-formal learning programmes are mostly organized keeping in mind the convenience of the organizers as well as the learners. Like formal education, measures are also taken to carry out both formative and summative assessment by mid-term review and final review (Sharma et al. 2017).

13.3 Importance of Creating a Positive Learning Environment

There is growing evidence that a positive learning environment increases student achievement. It also contributes to learning and helps in building strong relationships between teachers and learners. A positive learning environment also provides a feeling of safety to students, staff and visitors. A good learning environment helps in building a culture of mutual trust and respect that engages the learners meaningfully in the task of learning. Besides that, it also supports a relationship between teaching and learning that helps in improving mental health and academic performance. If you could create a learning environment, which is culturally and linguistically diverse, it results in stronger connections between each student and teacher. Therefore, a positive learning environment does not only help a learner to perform better cognitively but also ensures a balanced development of his/her personality (Tucker et al. 2003).

13.4 Bedside as a Learning Environment

Bedside teaching (BST) has been defined as, 'a part of clinical rounds where both student and instructor attends the patient's bedside to discuss the case and/or demonstrate a clinical procedure'. Garout et al. (2016) say that bedside teaching helps the students understand the doctor's relationship with the patient better and provides them with first-hand experience on supervised instruction, interviewing a patient, physical examination, communication and counselling.

BST is a fundamental component of clinical training and an essential tool in the creation of a competent physician. Sir William Osler, one of Canada's most renowned physicians who introduced BST to medical education in 1892, described that medical education needed to be taught at the bedside (LaCombe 1997; Peters and Ten Cate 2014). BST allows the physician and patient to interact at the bedside as it is through this physician-patient interaction process that the medical students and residents are simultaneously afforded the opportunity to learn clinical skills, clinical reasoning, physician-patient communication, empathy and professionalism. Clinical teaching involving patients is enriched by these visual, auditory and tactile experiences. The BST learning triad comprises patients, students and tutors. All three must be present for BST to occur and it must occur within a clinical environment. Each individual member tends to bring his or her own value to the learning triad. For example, the student brings medical knowledge and the eagerness to learn; the tutor brings depth of knowledge, mentorship and willingness to help the student learn and make connections; and finally, the patient brings relevant clinical issues to the forefront that allow the student to learn. An effective learning environment requires all three groups to work together in the learning triad. The ultimate solution is incorporating more bedside teaching into student timetables and giving doctors more protected teaching time. Crumlish et al. (2009) and Doumouras et al. (2015) claim that several senior medical students and medical residents believe BST to be a highly valuable yet underutilized practice.

13.5 Clinical Skills Laboratory

The main objective of the medical curriculum is to provide medical students with knowledge, skills and attitudes required for their practice. A decade ago, the UK Medical Council issued a report called 'Tomorrow's Doctors' (GMC 2003)which called for the reduction in the factual content of the medical course with the promotion of problem-based, self-dedicated learning. This report was the basis for a move towards an extensive reform of the medical and nursing curricula. The new reformed curricula enhanced the integrated medical teaching and emphasized the teaching and learning of clinical skills. However, Al-Elq (2007) and Tucker et al. (2003) report that there were still concerns about the standards and appropriateness of the skills of new medical graduates. The emergence of clinical skills laboratories (CSLs) in the medical education of many medical and nursing schools was caused by the changes in the teaching and learning methods, the radical changes in the healthcare delivery and the rapid growth of technology which challenged the traditional way of clinical skills development.

Clinical skills laboratories are educational facilities that benefit the undergraduate and postgraduate medical students and medical staff. They provide a safe and protected environment in which the learner can practise clinical skills before using them in real clinical settings. These skills laboratories help to ensure that all students acquire the necessary techniques and are properly assessed before practising on real patients. In addition, they support the acquisition, maintenance and enhancement of the clinical skills of students in the healthcare profession. Al-Yousuf (2004) elucidates that the term 'clinical skills' involves history-taking, physical examination, clinical investigations, using diagnostic reasoning, procedural perfection, effective communication, teamwork and professionalism.

Medical schools and postgraduate centres have gone to considerable lengths to create educational facilities dedicated to the teaching of clinical skills. The first CSL was established in Maastricht, the Netherlands, Limburg University, 1976. Since then, many medical schools and educational institutions have integrated CSLs into their curricula. In general, the exact nature of the skill taught is usually determined by the local logistical and educational requirements. With advances in technology and the changes in teaching methodology, the list of skills that are taught and learnt in the CSLs has grown longer. Because of the variety of these skills, it is important to define them and determine the level of competence required at each institution. Bradley and Postlethwaite (2003) say that it is for this reason that many CSLs involve curriculum development committees and undergraduate and postgraduate faculty members in their planning process.

13.6 Skills that Can Be Taught and Learnt in Clinical Skills Laboratory

Investigational skills—Test selection and data interpretation.
Patient management.
Resuscitation procedure and techniques.
Clinical reasoning and critical appraisal.
Teaching and learning methodology.
Presentation skill.
Communication skill.
Information and communication technology (ICT).
Prescribing skill.
Documentation.
Clinical and legal consideration.
Health safety and manual handling.
Attitudinal awareness and professionalism.
Administrative, economic and organization skills.
Leadership.
Teamwork and interprofessional skills learning.

13.7 Setting the Educational Environment

In setting up a clinical skill facility, it is important to follow the modern educational theory in the development and delivery of the programme. The development of communication skills is a crucial area of focus for CSLs. Bradley and Postlethwaite

(2003) say that as the proper application of clinical skills require the integration of technical clinical skills and communication skills, the better name for those laboratories would be clinical and communication skills centres or units.

Student-centred, integrated, problem-based and self-directed learning educational strategies including multi-profession, community-oriented or outcome-based education can be adapted in CSLs. Moreover, methods of learning may include a small group, a large group, real, standardized and simulated patients or role play. Audio and video recording is important especially in the development of communication skills.

Clinical skills laboratories vary in location, shape and site depending upon the availability of space and resources. Clinical skills laboratories may consist of a large open space for seminars and several small side rooms for interviews. It may also include a variety of clinical settings such as general practice consulting rooms, procedural skills rooms, accident and emergency cubicles with an intensive care unit and a place for simulators. Storage areas and offices are important especially for the teachers and support staff. In order to suit the varying lessons, it is necessary that the available space is kept fluid for possible rearrangement. Al-Yousuf (2004) and Bradley and Postlethwaite (2003) think that it is essential that a clinical skills facility provides a sense of real clinical environment.

13.8 Simulation-Based Learning Environments in Medical Education

Al-Elq (2010) says that simulation-based learning environments allow students to interact with patients, diagnostic laboratory procedures and patient data in a virtual environment and are designed to improve the quality of medical education.

The simulation-based learning environments have proved to increase students' learning, intrinsic motivation and self-efficacy and increased the perceived relevance of medical educational activities. Simulations can help future generations of doctors transfer new understanding of disease mechanisms gained in virtual laboratory settings into everyday clinical practice.

Physical simulations like training emergency care workers to use mannequins have been used widely for many years. The emergence of digital simulation technologies now provides innovative ways for conveying medical knowledge by using case stories in highly realistic clinical scenarios. These simulations enable learners to see and interact with representations of natural phenomena that would otherwise be impossible to observe. According to Cant and Cooper (2010), for advancement in the field of education, it is essential to combine learning and assessment, and they believe that simulations have the potential to do it.

Meta-analyses have found that deliberate practice through simulations is an efficient way to acquire medical and clinical expertise. Many researchers have demonstrated the benefits of simulation technology over traditional lectures in improving specific surgical technical skills, cardiovascular examination skills and acquisition and retention of knowledge. Simulations are also effective in enhancing interpersonal and communication skills in healthcare professionals. Therefore, DeCaporale-Ryan et al. (2016) say that simulation technology helps improve engagement and motivation for learning and is better than the traditional approaches in skills development.

Simulation is an important component of the clinical and communication skills centres. Simulators can be classified into four types:

1. A part-time trainer: training model which represents part of the body or structure that can be used alone or can be attached to simulated patients for simultaneous technical and communication skills development.
2. A computer-based system which can be in the form of (a) multimedia programme using audio and video systems, (b) interactive systems which provide the users with clinical variables that can be manipulated to provide feedback on the decisions and actions and (c) virtual reality that creates environments or objects such as computer-generated imaging that replicate kinaesthetic and tactile perception.
3. Simulated patients and environments: simulated patients can be professional actors trained to present history and sometimes mimic physical signs or can be trained patients. Both can be used as standardized patients. Creation of simulated environment is common in CSLs.
4. Integrated simulators: these simulators combine mannequins with advanced computer controls that can be adjusted to provide various physiological parameter outputs.

Adequate staffing is an essential aspect playing a major role in the success of CSLs. Both teaching and support staff should be selected carefully. Teaching staff can be full-time, part-time and seasonal or peripatetic clinical skills teachers. The support staff usually includes administrators, patient coordinators, a secretary and technicians. Finally, depending on its setting, CSLs can be used for teaching and learning at both undergraduate and postgraduate levels. Cant and Cooper (2010) say that medical students, nursing students and dentistry and applied medical science students can also make use of CSLs.

13.9 Guidelines for Successful Implementation

For many medical schools, the high cost of the facility and equipment and the need for continuous update and maintenance are a major barrier to the incorporation of CSLs in their curriculum. Many teaching staff who are strong believers of bedside clinical teaching may resist the change. Al-Elq (2007) also says that in addition to this, the planning skills centres involve a variety of stakeholders and users, some of whom may not be enthusiastic for change. Since CSLs are costly, it is important to ensure that the outcome is justifiable so that investors can be persuaded. Clinical skills laboratories should be designed to support the intended learning outcome and to form an integral part of the overall curriculum. The development of clinical skills should be integrated into the communication skills programme and other parts of the curricula, to avoid reverting to formal method of education. To be successful, clinical skills units need to be flexible in design and schedule and need to be within or near the medical schools. Al-Yousuf (2004), Joseph et al. (2015) and Lateef (2010) strongly insist that as far as possible, the environment and the clinical space should try to mimic the conditions of real practice.

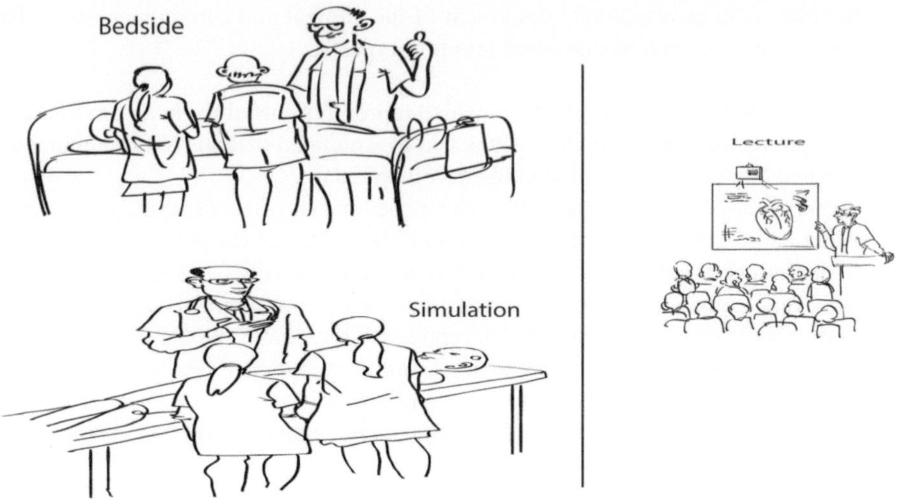

Fig. 13.2 Educational environment—as it should be

Conclusion

In conclusion, in today's world with the rapid changes in the medical education and the fast-paced technological development, environment plays a vital role for the acquisition of clinical skills and other professional characteristics. Many clinical skills can be learnt and taught in ideal environments and can be assessed using appropriate tools. Hence, the effectiveness of any learning environment depends on the factors like identifying the learning needs of the learners, availability and accessibility of the learning resources, setting up of learning spaces and availability of trained faculty and skilled trainers.

References

Al-Elq AH (2007) Medicine and clinical skills laboratories. J Family Community Med 14:59–63

Al-Elq AH (2010) Simulation-based medical teaching and learning. J Family Community Med 17:35–40. https://doi.org/10.4103/1319-1683.68787

Al-Yousuf NH (2004) The clinical skills laboratory as a learning tool for medical students and health professionals. Saudi Med J 25:549–551

Bradley P, Postlethwaite K (2003) Setting up a clinical skills learning facility. Med Educ 37(Suppl 1):6–13

Cant RP, Cooper SJ (2010) Simulation-based learning in nurse education: systematic review. J Adv Nurs 66:3–15. https://doi.org/10.1111/j.1365-2648.2009.05240.x

Colliver JA (2002) Educational theory and medical education practice: a cautionary note for medical school faculty. Acad Med J Assoc Am Med Coll 77:1217–1220

Crumlish CM, Yialamas MA, McMahon GT (2009) Quantification of bedside teaching by an academic hospitalist group. J Hosp Med 4:304–307. https://doi.org/10.1002/jhm.540

DeCaporale-Ryan LN, Dadiz R, Peyre SE (2016) Simulation-based learning: from theory to practice. Fam Syst Health 34:159–162. https://doi.org/10.1037/fsh0000203

Doumouras A, Rush R, Campbell A, Taylor D (2015) Peer-assisted bedside teaching rounds. Clin Teach 12:197–202. https://doi.org/10.1111/tct.12296

Garout M, Nuqali A, Alhazmi A, Almoallim H (2016) Bedside teaching: an underutilized tool in medical education. Int J Med Educ 7:261–262. https://doi.org/10.5116/ijme.5780.bdba

General Medical Council. Tomorrow's Doctors. London: GMC 2003.

Haddock KS (1994) A precepted leadership course based on Bandura's social learning theory. Nursingconnections 7:55–61

Hartzell JD (2007) Adult learning theory in medical education. Am J Med 120:e11. https://doi.org/10.1016/j.amjmed.2006.10.024

Hutchinson L (2003) Educational environment. BMJ 326:810–812. https://doi.org/10.1136/bmj.326.7393.810

Joseph N, Nelliyanil M, Jindal S, Utkarsha, Abraham A, Alok Y, Srivastava N, Lankeshwar S (2015) Perception of simulation-based learning among medical students in South India. Ann Med Health Sci Res 5:247–252. https://doi.org/10.4103/2141-9248.160186

Kaufman DM (2003) Applying educational theory in practice. BMJ 326:213–216

LaCombe MA (1997) On bedside teaching. Ann Intern Med 126:217–220

Lateef F (2010) Simulation-based learning: just like the real thing. J Emerg Trauma Shock 3:348–352. https://doi.org/10.4103/0974-2700.70743

Peters M, Ten Cate O (2014) Bedside teaching in medical education: a literature review. Perspect Med Educ 3:76–88. https://doi.org/10.1007/s40037-013-0083-y

Remmen R (1998) Unsatisfactory basic skills performance by students in traditional medical curricula. Med Teach 20:579–582. https://doi.org/10.1080/01421599880328

Sharma CB, Pathak A, Sinha A (2017) Unit-8 Learning Enviornment: Meaning and Scope. IGNOU.

Spencer J (2003) Learning and teaching in the clinical environment. BMJ 326:591–594. https://doi.org/10.1136/bmj.326.7389.591

Stewart TJ (2006) Learning environments in medical education. Med Teach 28:387–389. https://doi.org/10.1080/01421590600727043

Taylor DCM, Hamdy H (2013) Adult learning theories: implications for learning and teaching in medical education: AMEE Guide No. 83. Med Teach 35:e1561–e1572. https://doi.org/10.3109/0142159X.2013.828153

Thomas A, Menon A, Boruff J, Rodriguez AM, Ahmed S (2014) Applications of social constructivist learning theories in knowledge translation for healthcare professionals: a scoping review. Implement Sci 9(54). https://doi.org/10.1186/1748-5908-9-54

Torre DM, Daley BJ, Sebastian JL, Elnicki DM (2006) Overview of current learning theories for medical educators. Am J Med 119:903–907. https://doi.org/10.1016/j.amjmed.2006.06.037

Tucker K, Wakefield A, Boggis C, Lawson M, Roberts T, Gooch J (2003) Learning together: clinical skills teaching for medical and nursing students. Med Educ 37:630–637

Wiskin C, Barrett M, Fruhstorfer B, Schmid ML (2018) Recommendations for undergraduate medical electives: a UK consensus statement. Med Educ 52:14–23. https://doi.org/10.1111/medu.13445

Yardley S, Teunissen PW, Dornan T (2012) Experiential learning: AMEE Guide No. 63. Med Teach 34:e102–e115. https://doi.org/10.3109/0142159X.2012.650741

Programme Evaluation

14

Objectives

1. To establish the meaning for programme evaluation.
2. To state the need for evaluation of educational programmes.
3. To provide a framework for evaluation of educational programmes.

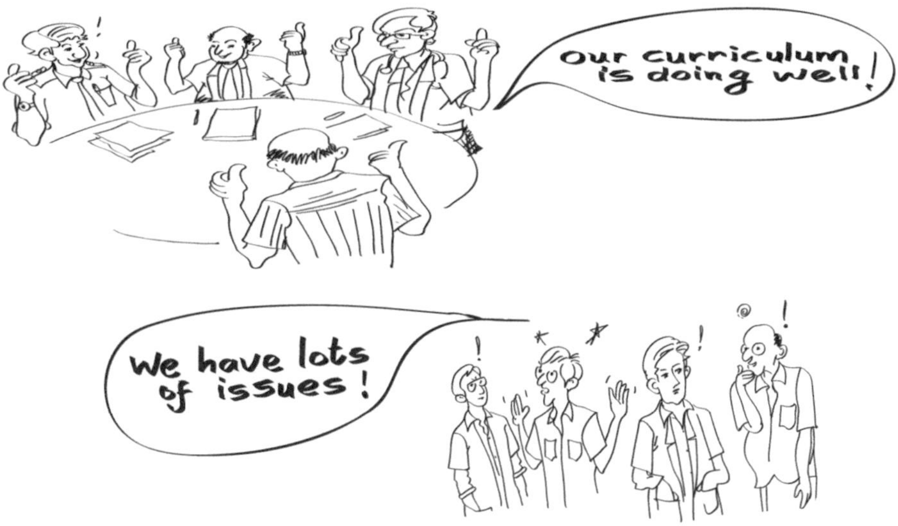

Fig. 14.1 Programme evaluation: not valued

Kadambari D et al., *Improving Discipline-Based Undergraduate Medical Curriculum*, https://doi.org/10.1007/978-981-13-1310-3_14

14.1 Introduction

Medical curriculum is a dynamic one which is intended to produce medical graduates with appropriate knowledge, attitude and skills of medicine keeping in mind the emerging healthcare needs of the society. Hence, the curriculum needs to be continuously reviewed to determine its quality and to understand how students perform as per the curricular objectives stated in the curriculum. A systematic and comprehensive programme evaluation is the means to understand whether the curriculum is achieving the stated goals. The evaluation process involves determining standards to assess the quality, collecting appropriate information and applying the standards to evaluate the effectiveness and value of the evaluation object. Curriculum evaluation system should ensure that the curriculum is appropriate for the proposed education that is intended to develop competent physicians. It should use appropriate tools to test the effectiveness of the program. It should inform the academic heads, its faculty and students about the effectiveness of the programme. Specific evaluation plan is needed to evaluate the components of the curriculum using appropriate evaluation mechanisms.

Educational programs are fundamentally about behavioural change, and programme evaluation is designed to determine the change. The programme evaluation should examine for both intended and unintended changes. Programme evaluation studies have been strongly influenced by reductionist theory, which attempts to isolate individual programme components to determine associations with outcomes. Educational programmes are complex, with multiple interactions among participants and the environment, such that system theory or complexity theory may be better suited to informing programme evaluation. The association between programme elements and outcomes may be non-linear—small changes in programme elements may lead to large changes in outcomes and vice versa. Educationists should always have an open mind to predict the outcome of an educational programme without limiting themselves to an incomplete view of the programme which is under evaluation. We should choose a programme evaluation model that allows us to examine for change in the programme and embraces the complexity of the educational process. According to Fitzpatrick et al. (2010), programme evaluation is defined as 'the identification, clarification, and application of defensible criteria to determine an evaluation object's value in relation to those criteria'. In broad terms, this process involves determining standards to assess the quality, collecting appropriate information and applying the standards to evaluate the effectiveness and value of the evaluation object. In broad terms programme evaluation is a systematic process to determine the worth, strength, sufficiency or allure of something with respect to specific criteria and goals. Vassar et al. (2010) believe that programme evaluation is the process of judging the worth of a programme and the judgement should be shaped by comparing the existing programme with the set criteria on what the programme should be.

14.2 Framework for Programme Evaluation

Prior to conducting a course evaluation, it is useful to consider a framework within which to situate one's work. The four guiding domains that guide the curriculum committee to evaluate any education programme are the following:

1. Why are we evaluating this programme? (Achievement of curriculum goals).
2. What are we going evaluate? (Educational process and outcomes).
3. Who is going to evaluate? (Self, peer, students).
4. When are we going to evaluate? (During the course, at the end of the course and after a long run) (Kirkpatrick and Kirkpatrick 2016).

This section provides the framework to evaluate the medical education programme advocated by Donald Kirkpatrick which is extensively employed to evaluate the effectiveness of educational programmes (Kirkpatrick and Kirkpatrick 2016; Reed 2011). Donald Kirkpatrick formulated the four levels of evaluation, and each level presents an order of steps to evaluate educational programmes. Reaction level evaluates the approach of the student towards the programme; learning level evaluates the knowledge achieved by the sample population having been exposed to the education; behaviour level measures how properly the knowledge achieved is put into use by trainees; results level measures how appropriately the major aim of the education is attained (Kirkpatrick and Kirkpatrick 2016).

14.3 Levels of Programme Evaluation

14.3.1 Level 1: Reaction

This evaluates the quality of instruction, quality of handouts and other learning resources and quality of facilities. All these are evaluated keeping in mind the learners' characteristics, learning environment and characteristics of learning materials. This is usually done by taking feedback from the learners at the end of any instruction or learning experience. They can be rated on a scale of 1–5 where 1 stands for not at all and 5 stands for very. Generally formed as a survey or questionnaire, participants hint this level as 'happy sheets' or 'feel-good measure', and an organized way as to participants' response to the programme could contain basic questions such as (Goldie 2006; Wilkes and Bligh 1999):

- Are the programme guidelines clear and communicated well?
- To what extent does the programme met your learning needs?
- How is it better than the previous programme or activity?
- What is your favourite part of the programme?
- Are there areas for improvement?

Kirkpatrick and Kirkpatrick (2016) and Schiekirka et al. (2015) state the aim of measuring reaction is to guarantee that participants are motivated and involved in learning. He shows the implementation guidelines of reaction level as in the following:

- Determine what you want to find out.
- Design a form that will quantify reactions.
- Encourage written comments and suggestions.
- Attain an immediate response rate of 100%.
- Seek honest reactions.
- Develop acceptable standards.
- Measure reactions against the standard and take appropriate action.
- Communicate the reactions as appropriate.

14.3.2 Level 2: Learning

This evaluates the students' demonstrable knowledge, attitude and skills at the end of the learning experience. This can be done by conducting tests before, during and after any learning experience. They can be rated on a scale of 1–5 where 1 stands for not at all and 5 stands for very.

We can evaluate if specific abilities or awareness levels have been transformed into more developed ones as a result of the programme, and some other measurable acquisitions contain the following as well (Cook 2010; Fitzpatrick et al. 2010; Goldie 2006; Vassar et al. 2010):

- Using formal, informal means of measuring the knowledge, attitude and psychomotor skills using appropriate tools.

The implementation guidelines referred by Kirkpatrick and Kirkpatrick (2016) for learning level are as follows:

- Use a control group, if feasible.
- Evaluate knowledge, skills or attitudes both before and after training.
- Use a paper and pencil test to measure knowledge and skills.
- Use a performance test to measure attitudes.
- Attain a response rate of 100%.
- Use the results of the evaluation to take appropriate action.

14.3.3 Level 3: Behaviour

Kirkpatrick's third level of evaluation is behaviour. This evaluates to what extent the students apply their knowledge, attitude and skills acquired during their education. Although learning has taken place, it doesn't mean that this learning transforms into new behaviour in real life (Kirkpatrick and Kirkpatrick 2016; Schiekirka et al. 2015;

Vassar et al. 2010). Behaviour evaluation suggests that learners apply the pre-learnt items afterwards and change their behaviours as a result, and this might be instantly or much time after the education process, based on the position (Haji et al. 2013; Vassar et al. 2010). Third level makes us conclude whether alterations in behaviour have happened as a result of the program, and also Kirkpatrick points out the necessity of having data on the first and the second levels to clarify the outcomes of the third-level evaluation (Tavakol et al. 2010). If the behaviour change does not appear, it is convenient to decide whether this is because of the participant's discontentment with the first level or lack of success in terms of the aims of the second level or whether the shortage of change in behaviour is because of some other reasons like a lack of desire, aid or opportunity. Implementation guidelines of this level are as follows (Kirkpatrick and Kirkpatrick 2016; Reed 2011):

- Use a control group, if feasible.
- Allow enough time for a change in behaviour to take place.
- Survey or interview one or more of the following groups: trainees, their bosses, their subordinates and others who often observe trainees' behaviour on the job.
- Choose an appropriate sampling.
- Repeat the evaluation at appropriate times.
- Consider the cost of evaluation versus the potential benefits.

14.3.4 Level 4: Results (Impact)

Results is the fourth level of evaluation in Kirkpatrick's Framework which evaluates the improved learning outcomes and ultimately healthcare team performance. Kirkpatrick and Kirkpatrick (2016) state that results level can be referred as to what stated outcomes occur as a consequence of the outcomes of the learning activity and following reinforcement. The fourth level or results level is the most challenging part to evaluate adequately, and this level describes results to contain 'What impact has the change produced on the organization?' (Cook 2010; Durning et al. 2007). The objective of Kirkpatrick's fourth-level evaluation is to determine organizational outcomes in terms of performance, developments and benefits as well (Khanipoor et al. 2017). The aim of the fourth level of evaluation is also to measure the influence of the arranged event on the institution's goals. This should obviously show the student's ability to perform more successfully as a result of the education conducted (Evaluating Educational Programs. ERIC Digest. nd; Fitzpatrick et al. 2010; Wilkes and Bligh 1999). Implementation guidelines for this level are as follows:

- Use a control group, if achievable.
- Allow enough time for results to be accomplished.
- Assess both pre and post training, if feasible.
- Repeat the assessment at appropriate point of time.
- Consider the cost of evaluation versus the potential benefits.
- Be happy with the confirmation if supreme evidence isn't conceivable to achieve.

14.4 Process Evaluation

Process evaluation determines whether programme activities have been implemented as intended.

14.4.1 Various Domains and Their Process of Evaluation

14.4.1.1 Domain

To find out whether the expected level of knowledge, attitude and skills is being acquired by the medical graduates in order to fulfil their competencies.

Method of Evaluation

- Gather students' opinion on their development in the campus and how well the curriculum has prepared them to enter the field of medicine.
- Periodically, check if the education system or curriculum is meeting up with the medical institutions' adopted list of requirement for the completion of course by the students.
- Evaluate the students' performance in internship programmes, annually.
- Check the students' progress even after they complete their course in the institution, either through their employers if they are working or through their facilitators, if they are pursuing their higher studies.

14.4.1.2 Domain

To keep in check whether the assessment and evaluation mechanisms are competency based.

Method of Evaluation

- Check whether all the competencies are fulfilled by the curriculum and through evaluation; make sure that the students get the most out of the curriculum.
- Review the categories of requirements to determine where each objective fits into the curriculum.
- Analyse course and internship reports to determine the extent to which education and evaluation is competency based.
- Make sure appropriate descriptors are being used for competencies.
- Check for changes in competencies and update/modify the competency list every 3–5 years.

14.4.1.3 Domain

To ensure that the clinical presentation model has been adopted by the curriculum committee as the primary mechanism for integrating basic and clinical science content.

Method of Evaluation

- To determine the progress made in the clinical presentation model, the evaluation subcommittee should be made to provide an annual report.

- To analyse the extent to which the clinical presentation model is being used, course and internship reports should be studied thoroughly.

14.4.1.4 Domain

To ensure that the students are able to learn independently as it is very essential for them in order to provide quality healthcare when they become physicians.

Method of Evaluation

- Gather students' opinion on the academic environment as to how it promotes their independent learning, and evaluate these reports. Find out from these reports, the specific items with which student independent learning can be assessed.
- Activities should be conducted to promote independent learning and course and clerkship reports should contain information about them.
- The educational programme should also provide students with an idea of the characteristics of an outstanding physician, the inclusion of which leads to the complete professional development of students.
- Also make use of a student's self-evaluation and peer evaluation for the assessment of one's development.

14.4.1.5 Domain

To teach students how effective healthcare delivery additionally requires the thoughtfulness regarding family and community context setting.

Method of Evaluation

- Check the curriculum to make sure that this particular topic is addressed formally in it.

14.4.1.6 Domain

To provide the students with a balanced variety of clinical settings which are very essential for the students in order to master the competencies.

Method of Evaluation

- Choose how many inpatient versus outpatient clinical training sites should be made use of and monitor them properly.
- Choose how much primary care versus specialty care training should be given to the students and also monitor the amount properly.

14.4.1.7 Domain

To make use of informatics to acquire and utilize students' information effectively.

Method of Evaluation

- Make sure the informatics plan is adopted by the curriculum committee, and check the progress of the plan, periodically.
- Evaluate the extent to which the students make use of informatics.
- Study what course and clerkships make use of activities conducted through informatics.
- Assess how urban students feel vs the rural through informatics.

14.4.1.8 Domain

To provide opportunities for students to discover new knowledge and solutions.

Method of Evaluation

- Assess every student's level of educational research and publications and encourage their progress.

14.4.1.9 Domain

To encourage students to work individually as well as in groups to promote healthcare delivery.

Method of Evaluation

- Determine the various group activities conducted throughout the colleges, departments and specialties.

14.4.1.10 Domain

To provide the students an accommodating situation, which cultivates regard, individual honesty, service orientation and a feeling of individual prosperity in order to promote their learning and professional development.

Method of Evaluation

- Make sure that the annual class surveys contain information about these issues and addresses them.
- Organize a critical incident report program.

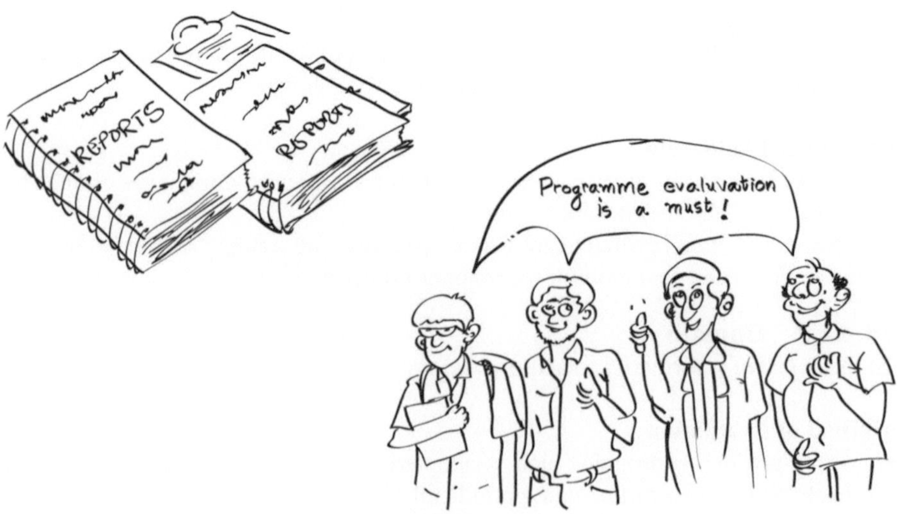

Fig. 14.2 Programme evaluation: being valued

Conclusion

Evaluation of the effectiveness of any educational programme is crucial for assessing the existing programmes and for designing future programmes that better address the needs of the learners and educational organizations. Programme evaluation should be more focused on answering the following: (1) How successful is the programme in preparing the participants for the stated programme goals? (2) What is the long-term impact of the programme on the participants' academic productivity and their professional development? (3) What directions the programme evaluation has for the organizers to take the programme further forward in all respects? Engaging in the process of evaluation of educational programmes would be invaluable for the growth and development of medical education.

References

Cook DA (2010) Twelve tips for evaluating educational programs. Med Teach 32(4):296–301. https://doi.org/10.3109/01421590903480121

Durning SJ, Hemmer P, Pangaro LN (2007) The structure of program evaluation: an approach for evaluating a course, clerkship, or components of a residency or fellowship training program. Teach Learn Med 19(3):308–318. https://doi.org/10.1080/10401330701366796

Evaluating Educational Programs. ERIC Digest (n.d.) Retrieved March 1, 2018, from https://www.ericdigests.org/pre-9217/programs.htm

Fitzpatrick JL, Sanders JR, Worthen BR (2010) Program evaluation: alternative approaches and practical guidelines, 4th edn. Pearson, Upper Saddle River, NJ

Goldie J (2006) AMEE Education Guide no. 29: evaluating educational programmes. Med Teach 28(3):210–224. https://doi.org/10.1080/01421590500271282

Haji F, Morin M-P, Parker K (2013) Rethinking programme evaluation in health professions education: beyond 'did it work?'. Med Educ 47(4):342–351. https://doi.org/10.1111/medu.12091

Khanipoor F, Amini M, Bazrafcan L (2017) Evaluation of educational program in the Master of Medical Education by Eisner's educational connoisseurship and criticism model. J Educ Health Promot 6:55. https://doi.org/10.4103/jehp.jehp_103_15

Kirkpatrick JD, Kirkpatrick WK (2016) Kirkpatrick's four levels of training evaluation, 1st edn. Association for Talent Development, Alexandria, VA

Reed DA (2011) Nimble approaches to curriculum evaluation in graduate medical education. J Grad Med Educ 3(2):264–266. https://doi.org/10.4300/JGME-D-11-00081.1

Schiekirka S, Feufel MA, Herrmann-Lingen C, Raupach T (2015) Evaluation in medical education: a topical review of target parameters, data collection tools and confounding factors. Ger Med Sci 13:Doc15. https://doi.org/10.3205/000219

Tavakol M, Gruppen LD, Torabi S (2010) Using evaluation research to improve medical education. Clin Teach 7(3):192–196. https://doi.org/10.1111/j.1743-498X.2010.00383.x

Vassar M, Wheeler DL, Davison M, Franklin J (2010) Program evaluation in medical education: an overview of the utilization-focused approach. J Educ Eval Health Prof 7:1. https://doi.org/10.3352/jeehp.2010.7.1

Wilkes M, Bligh J (1999) Evaluating educational interventions. BMJ 318(7193):1269–1272

MIX
Papier aus verantwortungsvollen Quellen
Paper from responsible sources
FSC® C105338

If you have any concerns about our products,
you can contact us on
ProductSafety@springernature.com

In case Publisher is established outside the EU,
the EU authorized representative is:
Springer Nature Customer Service Center GmbH
Europaplatz 3, 69115 Heidelberg, Germany

Printed by Libri Plureos GmbH
in Hamburg, Germany